low vision assessment

eye essentials

low vision assessment

Jane Macnaughton MCOptom
City University, London, UK
Director of Clearview Training, Leicestershire, UK

SERIES EDITORS
Sandip Doshi PhD, MCOptom
Optometrist in private practice, Hove, East Sussex, UK
Examiner, College of Optometrists, London, UK
Formerly Clinical Editor, Optician

William Harvey MCOptom
Visiting Clinician and Director of Visual Impairment Clinic,
City University, London, UK
Professional Programme Tutor for Boots Opticians Ltd
Clinical Editor, Optician, Reed Business Information, Sutton, UK
Examiner and Assessor, College of Optometrists, London, UK

First published 2005
Reprinted 2009

ISBN 0 7506 8854 8

British Library Cataloguing in Publication Data
A catalogue record for this book is available from the British Library.

Library of Congress Cataloging in Publication Data
A catalog record for this book is available from the Library of Congress.

Note

Knowledge and best practice in this field are constantly changing. As new research and experience broaden our knowledge, changes in practice, treatment and drug therapy may become necessary or appropriate. Readers are advised to check the most current information provided (i) on procedures featured or (ii) by the manufacturer of each product to be administered, to verify the recommended dose or formula, the method and duration of administration, and contraindications. It is the responsibility of the practitioner, relying on their own experience and knowledge of the patient, to make diagnoses, to determine dosages and the best treatment for each individual patient, and to take all appropriate safety precautions. To the fullest extent of the law, neither the publisher nor the editors assumes any liability for any injury and/or damage to persons or property arising from this publication.

Contents

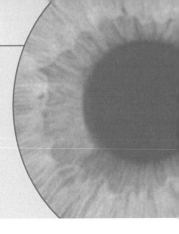

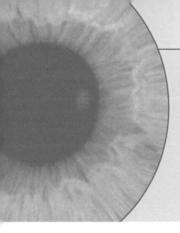

Acknowledgments

I would like to thank Bill Harvey for kindly contributing Chapter 8, regarding the psychology of visual impairment, and for the diagrams included in Chapter 5.

I would also like to thank Colin Longhurst of City University and Mark Silver of Visionary Imaging for their help with a number of the photographs included in Chapters 4, 5 and 6.

In addition I would like to extend a huge thank you to Dave Edgar for endless opportunity and to Janet Silver for putting me there in the first place.

This book is dedicated to Alexander, Callum and David.

Jane Macnaughton

Foreword

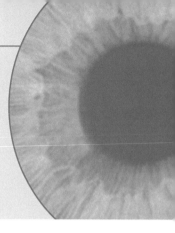

Eye Essentials is a series of books intended to cover
the core skills required by the eye care practitioner in general
and/or specialized practice. It consists of books covering a wide
range of topics, ranging from: routine eye examination to
assessment and management of low vision; assessment and
investigative techniques to digital imaging; case reports and
law to contact lenses.

Authors known for their interest and expertise in their
particular subject have contributed books to this series. The
reader will know many of them, as they have published widely
within their respective fields. Each author has addressed key
topics in their subject in a practical rather than theoretical
approach, hence each book has a particular relevance to
everyday practice.

Each book follows a similar format and has been designed
to enable the reader to ascertain information easily and
quickly. Each chapter has been produced in a user-friendly
format, thus providing the reader with a rapid-reference
book that is easy to use in the consulting room or in the
practitioner's free time.

Optometry and dispensing optics are continually developing
professions, with the emphasis in each being redefined as we
learn more from research and as technology stamps its mark.
The *Eye Essentials* series is particularly relevant to the
practitioner's requirements and, as such, will appeal to students,

graduates sitting professional examinations and qualified practitioners alike. We hope you enjoy reading these books as much as we have enjoyed producing them.

Sandip Doshi
Bill Harvey

Introduction

Introduction: provision of low vision aids

Approximately 70% of people included on the Blind and Partial Sight Registers in the United Kingdom are over 75 years of age (see Figure on opposite page). Macular degeneration is the most common cause, accounting for approximately half of registered cases.[1] With the management of systemic disease improving, it is expected that the number of elderly within our population is set to rise even further. The Department of Health has estimated that the total number of visually impaired is set to rise by 25% in the next 20 years.[2] This will undoubtedly have the effect of a greater demand for services for visually impaired people, which will include the provision of low vision aids.

It has been well known that for some time the provision of services for the visually impaired in the UK has been patchy.[2] As a result, a report published in 1999 by the Low Vision Consensus Group, *Recommendations for future service delivery in the United Kingdom*[3], proposed a national framework for low vision services, including the provision of low vision aids. The report emphasized the integration of relative disciplines, and the development of Low Vision Services Committees to coordinate the planning and monitoring of local and national services.

Following publication of the Consensus Group report, the College of Optometrists followed with a document entitled *Framework for a Multidisciplinary Approach to Low Vision*.[4] The aim of this document was to increase the level of optometric involvement in the provision of such low vision services. The document recognized the benefits of the multidisciplinary approach in which many professional groups work together as a team to provide an improved service to the visually impaired with the optometrist being an equal and integral member of this team. The document included input from members of the national Low Vision Implementation Group, established following publication of the Consensus Group report. This Group involves not only other professionals, but also lay members, many of whom are service users.

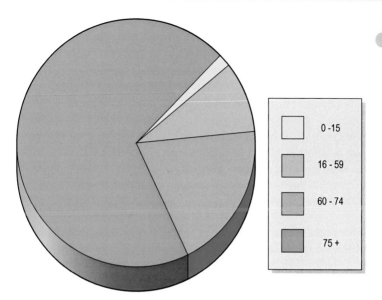

☐	0 -15
☐	16 - 59
☐	60 - 74
☐	75 +

Distribution of blindness and partial sight by age: UK[1]

Since publication of the documents, many such low vision groups have now become established throughout the UK.

A large proportion of low vision aids is prescribed through the hospital eye service (HES). The number of specialized clinics and experienced low vision practitioners are still too few to cover adequately the current estimated number of visually impaired people within the community. However, several research studies have indicated that the number of patients referred to hospital low vision clinics could be significantly reduced. It has been suggested that approximately 10–15% of patients attending hospital low vision clinics need a simple +4.00 Diopter addition and advice on lighting and available services for the visually impaired. This percentage increases further when we take into consideration that the majority of low vision aids dispensed from hospital low vision clinics are simple hand and stand magnifiers. With appropriate support, many of these patients could be comfortably managed within the General Ophthalmic Service.

In recognition of the importance of optometrists in low vision management in the community, both in terms of the skill set and accessibility, the government has designated low vision as one of the national eyecare pathways (along with cataract, macular degeneration and glaucoma) for which local primary care trusts are expected to develop dedicated schemes. As these develop with the help of increased funding and greater interprofessional integration, it is hoped that the fragmented provision of low vision services will eventually become a thing of the past.

Optometrists and dispensing opticians are in a strong position to provide low vision aids to patients through the General Ophthalmic Service. Twenty years ago it was estimated that only one-third of registered blind and partially sighted people had a low vision assessment and that at least half of those who had missed out would have benefited, had the opportunity arisen. As there are many visually impaired people who fall below the criteria for hospital referral the service has been very severely lacking.

As practitioners we can both recognize and assess a disease process. However, what we as individuals are unable to do is fully comprehend the impact the impairment will have upon a patient's way of life and how it affects their ability to live in a sighted world. Nevertheless, we are in a very strong position to provide a service to our visually impaired patients. Currently, there are too few practitioners willing to become involved in this area of clinical practice, and it is a sadly underused area of our expertise. Indeed, the limited number of low vision clinics and the scarcity of practitioners with low vision expertise is also a major reason why so many visually impaired people function below their true visual capacity.

Refraction and a basic understanding of the optics of low vision devices and magnifiers are essential if we are to have a thorough approach to prescribing magnification to our patients. Hopefully, this guide will bring a few more practitioners into a thoroughly rewarding area of clinical practice and to provide a more comprehensive approach to the patients we see daily within our practices.

The purpose of this book, therefore, is to produce a simplified key-facts guide for the practitioner who wishes to work with visually impaired patients on an occasional basis, with the emphasis on working with the elderly. Chapters are included on the younger populations, although the emphasis here is on advice and information, such as working with such groups often requires a multidisciplinary approach and specific expertise, more readily available within the hospital setting. As this book is primarily aimed at those beginning to gain experience in this area of optometry, Snellen notation is used throughout, as this is likely to be the acuity notation most familiar to the reader. It is important to remember, however, that logMAR notation is the norm in most low vision situations for reasons explained in Chapter 3.

A list of useful Internet sites is given towards the end of this book. Ray diagrams and core optics of devices are only covered when such detail is necessary and will help in practice. Indeed, it is assumed that the practitioner will have some basic knowledge of such.

VIPs, patients, clients or users?

Not all VIPs are Visually Impaired People, but all visually impaired people are VIPs. In hospital and general ophthalmic practice, the majority of optometrists and dispensing opticians will use the term 'patients'. Low vision practitioners of all backgrounds may use the term 'clients' or 'service users' and those with low vision will often describe themselves as 'users'. In fact, there are several names used in the work of low vision. For convenience, the term 'patient' will be used throughout this text with no intended partiality.

1

Definitions, certification and registration

Terminology

'A person with low vision is someone who has an impairment of visual function for whom full remediation is not possible by conventional spectacles, contact lenses or medical intervention and which causes restriction in that person's everyday life.' (Low Vision Consensus Group, 1999)[3]

Definitions. Why do we have them? As a society that is so keen to have everything and everyone 'labeled up', and put in the right box, why do we still have a need to give an awkward name to a person who is clearly a sufferer of a misfortune many of us still have difficulty confronting?

Both practitioners and patients need to use common and appropriate definitions so that we can all talk the same language. Correct terminology may act to segregate but it is also in the patient's favor to have their problem defined and recognized. Being appropriately 'certified' assists in ensuring protection and allows for a greater access to advice and information. Secondly, a patient's entitlements and rights will change when they have been put into the correct 'box' whether we agree with it or not.

A patient may be certified as blind or severely sight impaired but may not be disabled by their condition. A visually impaired person whose sight is not 'bad enough' for certification purposes may indeed be handicapped. What is most important (particularly from the patient's perspective) is for us all to understand why we have definitions in the first place.

World Health Organization definitions

WHO definition of low vision, 1993

'A person with low vision is one who has impairment of visual functioning even after treatment and/or standard refractive correction and has a visual acuity of less than 6/18 to light perception, or a visual field of less than 10° from the point of fixation, but who uses, or is potentially able to use, vision for the planning and/or execution of a task.'

ICF: The International Classification of Functioning, Disability and Health[5]

The World Health Organization first published a trial document in 1980 called the International Classification of Impairment, Disability and Handicap[6] (ICIDH). The purpose of the document was to provide a unified language and standard framework for the description of health and health-related states. The document was eventually finalized in 2000 as the ICF, the International Classification of Functioning, Disability and Health. It is often referred to as the ICIDH2.

The ICF belongs to the family of international classifications developed by the WHO for application of various aspects of health.[5] It is the WHO's framework for measuring health and disability at both individual and population levels, providing us with exceptionally broad and yet accurate tools to understand the health of a population and how the individual and his environment interacts. The ICF further provides the framework for health services, by measuring health outcomes to monitor and assess the effectiveness of health interventions. It meets the urgent demand for instruments to measure the performance of health interventions and health systems.[7]

Below are the definitions of Impairment, Disability and Handicap as outlined in the original document, the ICIDH (1980).

Impairment

'Any loss or abnormality of a psychological, physiological or anatomical structure or function.'

The term impairment refers to the functional consequence of a disease or disorder. In visual terms it refers to the physical loss experienced by the patient. The most common form of impairment would be a reduction in visual acuity; other impairments include, for example, a loss of visual field, color vision or contrast sensitivity.

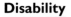

Disability

> *'Any restriction or inability (resulting from an impairment) to perform an activity in the manner or within the range considered normal for a human being.'*

When the impairment impacts on the ability to perform certain tasks, then the patient may be described as having a disability. A reduction in near acuity is one of the most significant visual impairments by which a patient can be disabled.

However, not all impairments will lead to a disability. A congenital color vision defect will have no impact on the ability to read small print, and a presbyope, who requires spectacles to read, may have a visual impairment but is no longer disabled by it when they put their spectacles on.

Handicap

> *'Any disadvantage for a given individual, resulting from an impairment or a disability, that limits or prevents the fulfilment of a role that is normal (depending upon age, sex and social and cultural factors) for that individual.'*

The use of the term handicap widens the context from the individual to the environment in which they function. An individual who is unable to read his printed bank statements may be handicapped by the loss of privacy. Similarly, the presbyopic tailor in an underdeveloped country who has no access to spectacles may no longer be able to work to feed his family.

The definition of handicap is the most controversial. In the UK, many health care professionals no longer use the term handicap. A patient may instead be described as being 'disabled by' aspects of the environment. Not all disabilities lead to handicaps. To some, the inability to read small print may be a nuisance, but to others it can be a major source of handicap. Thus, a person will not be handicapped if the impairment or disability does not stop them from doing what they want to do: it either has not affected the way in which they live, or that they have overcome the consequences of the disability.

Careful questioning within the low vision assessment will determine such levels of disability or handicap. Therefore, in order to decide whether a person has, or does not have, a handicap, we have to look at their lifestyle, and to find out in which of these areas he or she is not integrated. But it is clearly not always a question of mental attitude. The following case example highlights this.

Case example John A: Retinitis pigmentosa

A young, single male is diagnosed with retinitis pigmentosa. His initial impairment is that of night blindness. The following is a list of everyday situations and how this patient described his situation:

- Night blindness (*the impairment*). Problems finding his way back to the taxi rank after a night out. His friends find him and give him a lift home.
- His friends arrange to meet him the next day in the cinema for an early evening showing and the sun is still shining when he makes his way. However, he arrives late and the film has already started. Due to problems with dark adaptation (*impairment*) he is unable to locate them inside the cinema theatre. He gives up, frustrated, and goes home.
- Further progression of the disease results in a gradual constriction of the visual field (*impairment*). He has difficulty finding his way around a supermarket and, feeling awkward, finds it necessary to enlist the help of a member of staff.

For many people the above examples are frustrating and do require a review of their lifestyle, some managing more than others. Most would consider the above situations a disability. The mobility problem in the supermarket could become a handicap if it stopped him from shopping for his weekly groceries, or indeed, stopped him from going out altogether.

Despite being diagnosed in his late teens, this patient was determined to become a surgeon. Now 40, and a father of three boys, he was forced to give up his surgical career. Instead he has become a full-time father, his GP wife now working full time.

He is unable to drive and relies on friends to pick the children up from school. It is easy to see that his impairment has handicapped him by cutting short his career and he is now unable to work in his designated field to support his family. Not only has his driver's licence been revoked but also he is unable to practice medicine. With a severe restriction in visual field and acuity, he prefers not to walk his three year old the few hundred yards to the park in case he loses him. With later stage development of the disease, he developed posterior subcapsular cataracts. Coupled together with less than a ten-degree field, working at the computer has also become an impossibility without the aid of synthetic speech. The above examples are more typical of a handicap.

Thankfully, he had been aware of his situation from an early age, his older brother also having been affected. Thus, he had made sufficient plans for the future and works occasionally as a lecturer, supported by excellent staff and equipment.

UK definitions for the purpose of certification

Many different definitions of visual impairment are used for the purpose of legislation throughout the world. In the UK, patients are either **certified** as severely sight impaired or sight impaired, before being included on a local authority or primary care trust **register**.

The Social Services Department, or local voluntary group acting on behalf of the Primary Care Trust, has a duty to maintain the register of people certified as blind or partially sighted.

Blind certification and the BD8 (1990)[8]
The BD8 (1990) was the 'Record of examination to certify a person as blind or partially sighted'. It did not take into consideration other physical or mental conditions. This document was used in England and Wales, and similar documents are used in Scotland (BP1)[9] and Northern Ireland (A655).[10] Definitions for the purpose of certification are similar on all three documents, although the BP1 and A655 request further information on the

patient's disabilities, which can be useful for rehabilitation purposes. However, the BP1 appears to be the only document that takes into consideration the patient's near acuity.

The Certificate of Vision Impairment

In November 2003 the BD8 was formally replaced by the Certificate of Vision Impairment (CVI 2003). This document is currently for England only (Fig. 1.1).

The new form is the result of consultation with a number of different parties, including service users, academics, the Association of Directors of Social Services, Department of Culture, Media and Sport, Department of Work and Pensions, Inland Revenue, National Assembly of Wales, Northern Ireland, optometrists, RNIB and various other voluntary organisations, Royal College of Ophthalmologists, Scottish Executive, social workers and specialist rehabilitation workers.[11]

The CVI performs the same function as BD8.[11] That is, it formally certifies someone as partially sighted or as blind (now using the preferred terminology 'sight impaired' or 'severely sight impaired', respectively) so that the local health authority can register him or her. Registration, although voluntary, enables access to various benefits, but access to social services is *not* dependent on registration. It also acts as a referral for a social care assessment if the person has not previously been brought to the attention of social services, as someone with needs arising from their visual impairment.

The aim of the new scheme is to decouple the formal process of registration from the initiation of an assessment of needs. However, both elements are still important and will continue.[12]

The focus of the CVI is in the delivery of information of benefits and services for users. Patients will, therefore, have a greater access to information and services from the time that a problem has been identified rather than having to wait for registration with the local authority. In addition, the CVI aims to accumulate a significant amount of epidemiological data that can be used in the planning of future services.[13]

Certificate of Vision Impairment (CVI 2003)

Certificate of a Person as
Sight Impaired / Partially Sighted or as
Severely Sight Impaired / Blind

Copies in confidence to:

[Hospital eye service to delete this text and replace with hospital logo and / or clinic contact details]

☐ Local council / Care trust
☐ Patient
☐ Patient's GP
☐ Hospital notes
☐ Epidemiological analysis (see current explanatory notes for instructions and address.)

Part 1: to be completed by a consultant ophthalmologist

A. Patient's details

Title and Surname	Address
Other names	
	Email
Date of birth	Daytime Tel.
Details of general practitioner Name Address Tel.	Details of local social services / agent Name Address Tel.

B. Visual function

Visual acuity (Snellen, LogMAR or functional assessment, e.g. hand movement or finger counting)	Right eye	Left eye
Unaided		
Best corrected		
Best corrected with both eyes		

Field of vision (Tick box if abnormal)		Low vision service (Tick one box)	
Total loss of visual field		Has been assessed	
Extensive loss of visual field (including hemianopia)		To be assessed	
Primary loss of peripheral field		Not relevant or the patient does not want an assessment	
Primary loss of central field			

Does sight vary markedly in different light levels?	☐	☐

Figure 1.1 The Certificate of Vision Impairment (CVI 2003)

Letter of Vision Impairment, or LVI (2003)

In addition to the CVI (2003), the Letter of Vision Impairment, or LVI, has been produced. This letter can be given to the patients by the optometrist to be used by those wishing to self-refer.

Referral of Vision Impaired patient, or RVI (2003)

This form allows a patient to be directly referred to social services in cases where treatment is not deemed necessary and may improve the speed of access to social services help.

Definition: severely sight impaired (blind)[14]

The National Assistance Act 1948 states that a person can be certified as blind if they are:

'so blind that they cannot perform any work for which eyesight is essential'. [National Assistance Act, Section 64(1)]

The test is whether a person cannot do *any work* for which eyesight is essential, not just his or her normal job or one particular job. Only the condition of the person's *eyesight* should be taken into account. Any other physical or mental condition should be ignored. The main condition to consider is what the person's *visual acuity* is. ('Visual Acuity is the best direct vision that can be obtained, with appropriate spectacle correction if necessary, with each eye separately, or with both eyes together if a person has both. Visual acuity is tested to Snellen's type.')

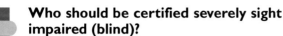
Who should be certified severely sight impaired (blind)?

People can be classified into three groups.

Group 1: People who are below 3/60 Snellen

Certify as blind:
Most people who have visual acuity below 3/60 Snellen.

Do not certify as blind:
People who have visual acuity of 1/18 Snellen unless they also have considerable restriction of visual field.

> In many cases it is better to test the person's vision at one meter. 1/18 Snellen indicates a slightly better acuity than 3/60 Snellen. But it may be better to specify 1/18 Snellen because the standard test types provide a line of letters, which a person who has a full acuity should read at 18 meters.

Group 2: People who are 3/60 but below 6/60 Snellen

Certify as blind:
People who have a significantly contracted field of vision.

Do not certify as blind:
People who have a visual defect for a long time and who do not have a very contracted field of vision. For example, people who have congenital nystagmus, albinism, myopia and other conditions like these.

Group 3: People who are 6/60 Snellen or above

Certify as blind:
People in this group who have a severely contracted field of vision especially if the contraction is in the lower part of the field.

Do not certify as blind:
People who are suffering from homonymous or bitemporal hemianopia who still have central visual acuity 6/18 Snellen or better.

Other points to consider

These points are important because it is more likely that the ophthalmologist will certify a person in the following circumstances:

1. How recently the person's eyesight has failed: a person whose eyesight has failed recently may find it more difficult to adapt than a person with the same visual acuity whose eyesight failed a long time ago. This applies particularly to people who are in Groups 2 and 3 above.
2. How old the person was when their eyesight failed: an elderly person whose eyesight has failed recently may find it more difficult to adapt than a younger person with the same defect. This applies particularly to people in Group 2 above.

Sight impaired (partially sighted)

There is no legal definition of partial sight. The guidelines are that a person can be certified as partially sighted if they are *substantially and permanently handicapped by defective vision caused by congenital defect or illness or injury.*

People who are certified as partially sighted are entitled to the same help from their local social services as people who are certified as blind. But they may not be able to get certain social security benefits and tax concessions that only people who are certified as blind can get.

Department of Health guidelines

Who should be certified partially sighted:

VA 3/60–6/60 with a full field.

VA up to 6/24 with a moderately contracted visual field, opacities in the media or aphakia.

VA 6/18 or even better if there is a gross field defect, e.g. hemianopia, or if there is marked contraction of the visual field, e.g. retinitis pigmentosa or glaucoma.

Other points to consider

1. Infants and young children who have congenital ocular abnormalities leading to visual defect are certified as partially sighted, unless they are obviously blind.

2. Children aged 4 and over are certified as blind or partially sighted according to the corrected binocular vision.

Purpose and process of certification and registration

The general purpose in maintaining a register of severely sight impaired and sight impaired is so that local authorities can plan the provision of services to those visually impaired people within the local community. Despite this, it is important to note that to gain access to many services, a patient does not always need to be certified or registered. Under Community Care Legislation (Community Care Act 1990), if a person is able to demonstrate a 'need' for a specific service, then the local authority has a duty to provide it.

However, several studies by the RNIB have shown that people who have been registered with the local authority are more aware of benefits and services compared to those who are not registered.

Nevertheless, registration is required when claiming for all financial benefits and is often mandatory for many travel concessions and for assistance from voluntary groups.

The decision to certify

The decision to certify is taken by a consultant ophthalmologist. In a few cases, the consultant may take the decision not to certify an eligible patient. This decision may be due to a number of reasons; most commonly, the patient may not be emotionally ready and may be going through an early phase of the grieving process. Thus, caution on the part of the practitioner must be given if he is to make suggestions concerning eligibility to a patient when some other party may be dealing with the process. Registration, if handled badly, can be devastating. However, if handled well, it can be a positive move and not the 'end of the road' as is often portrayed.

Transferring and retaining the CVI

The patient will sign the certification document and therefore has agreed for a copy of the document to be forwarded to:

1. The Primary Care Trust/local authority for inclusion on the local register.
2. The GP.
3. The Office of National Statistics.

A copy of the CVI should be forwarded to the patient's GP and local authority within five working days of its completion. Notification may be additionally forwarded to:

4. Department of Employment for those persons of working age seeking employment.
5. DSS in the case of persons receiving income support.

What happens next?
In accordance with Progress in Sight, the Association of Directors of Social Services National Standards, on receipt of the CVI, the patient's social services department (or its agents) should contact the person and arrange for the following:

1. The social services team will organize a home visit to consider the patient's individual needs and to discuss individual entitlements, both national and local.
2. Their inclusion on the local authority's register (with the person's consent) and for them to be issued with a standardized registration card. The date of registration is taken to be the date that the ophthalmologist signed the certification document.

The CVI is an important source of information for health authority services and if a person moves to another area, it should be transferred to the person's new local social services. This will avoid the need for recertification.

The social services copy of the form should be kept until transferred to another authority or until there is evidence that the person is deceased.

What if it all goes wrong?

If, for some reason, a patient's form goes missing or perhaps he or she has not heard from the local authority, then the first step would be to contact the local authority directly. Most authorities will have a time frame during which the newly registered patient will be contacted.

If the patient is unhappy with the outcome of certification, he or she is also entitled to a second opinion from another consultant ophthalmologist. The patient would be first directed to his or her GP to initiate this.

In Wales, a separate system exists, and the patient is directed to the Ophthalmic Referee Service, run by the Wales Council for the Blind.

2
Epidemiology and causes of blindness and low vision

World statistics

It is estimated that 180 million people worldwide are visually impaired, with 50 million people bilaterally blind (less than 3/60 in the better seeing eye). Ninety percent of the world's blind live in the developing countries, 60% of which reside in sub-Saharan Africa, China and India.[15]

Approximately 50% of the world's blind suffer from cataract. Other prevailing conditions include glaucoma, trachoma, onchocerciasis and number of childhood blindness diseases (Fig. 2.1). According to World Health Organization (WHO) estimates, about 80% of global blindness is avoidable: either it results from the conditions that could have been prevented or controlled if the available knowledge and interventions had been timely applied (e.g. trachoma and onchocerciasis) or it can be successfully treated with the sight restored (e.g. cataract).[16]

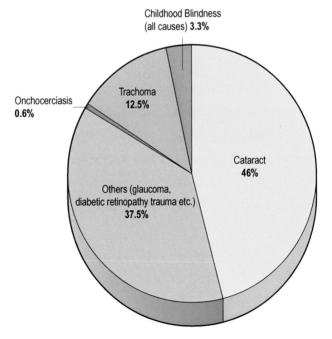

Figure 2.1 Global causes of blindness

Visual impairment is, therefore, most common in the developing countries. In Africa, about one in every hundred people are blind whereas in the better developed parts of Europe the prevalence of blindness is 0.33 per 1000.[17] The WHO estimates that cataract and refractive error account for 60% of global blindness with the remaining 40% split between focal diseases (occurring in focal clusters in the world), problem diseases that are becoming increasingly important as countries become more developed, and degenerative diseases. Degenerative diseases like age-related macular degeneration account for 10% of the total and the WHO estimates that the global figure for people blind with macular degeneration is 3 million (6%). Uncorrected ametropia has not been included here, but represents a major cause of global preventable visual impairment.

VISION 2020 The Right to Sight: a global initiative for the elimination of avoidable blindness[16]

It is predicted that the number of blind people will increase dramatically over the next 20 years to an estimated 75 million by 2020. In order to make a concerted worldwide effort to reduce global blindness, the WHO and a task force of international non-governmental organizations jointly prepared and launched a common agenda for global action, known as **Vision 2020**.

Vision 2020 is based on the concept of a broad coalition of all the organizations, which collaborate with the WHO in the prevention of blindness and eye care delivery, with the objective of eliminating avoidable blindness as a public health problem by the year 2020. These organizations will also jointly work to mitigate the implications of blindness in developmental, social, economic and quality-of-life terms.

In fully developed countries, macular degeneration accounts for half of blindness, with glaucoma and diabetic retinopathy causing a large proportion of the other half. Despite being avoidable, the management of untreated cataract and uncorrected refractive error requires considerable input from health care professionals, although these conditions have less significance in overall statistics of registerable blindness.

In developing countries, macular degeneration is not recognized as a significant cause of visual impairment largely because life expectancy is too short to be at risk of the disease. It is only likely to emerge as important as life expectancy increases.[17]

UK statistics

A recent study found that one in eight people over the age of 90 are visually impaired due to macular degeneration,[18] estimating that there are currently 182,000 individuals with vision in their best eye reduced to 6/18 or less. Blind registration data at least for the elderly, and particularly for age-related macular degeneration (ARMD), are probably better than previously thought. The last complete analysis 5 years ago[19] indicated that in half of all 65 year olds registered blind or partially sighted the cause is ARMD (Fig. 2.2).

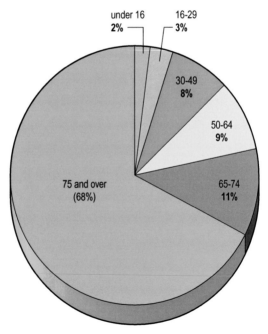

under 16
2%

16-29
3%

30-49
8%

50-64
9%

75 and over
(68%)

65-74
11%

Figure 2.2 Age distribution of visual impairment

There are as many people registered blind from ARMD as from glaucoma and diabetic retinopathy.[17,18] However, there are inherent biases with registration data; people with ARMD are more likely to be registered than those with diabetic retinopathy or glaucoma. Studies indicate that it is less likely that ophthalmologists will put patients under active treatment on the register. In the case of ARMD, because there have been so few treatment options until recently, the only help clinicians can offer is completion of the registration form.[17]

Registration statistics

It is widely agreed that the registration statistics are not a true representation of those with a visual impairment (Table 2.1). In 1995 the RNIB[1] concluded that, although the number of people registered both blind and partially sighted was 320,000, the real figure was estimated to be almost four times that amount. The number increases yet again if we take into account those whose sight is not within certification criteria, but who can be disabled by even a mild degree of visual impairment.

England

The publication SSDA 902[22] contains detailed statistics on persons registered with Councils with Social Services Responsibilities

Table 2.1 **Registered blind and partially sighted people: year ending 31 March 2003**

	Total number of people registered blind	Total number of people registered PS
England	156,675	155,230
Wales	9902	9905
Scotland[20]	23,557	14,443
N. Ireland (1995)[1,21]	Blind and partial sight total 5321	

(CSSRs) in England as being blind or partially sighted (Table 2.2). Councils compile the data from the triennial return SSDA 902 submitted to the Department of Health.

Main findings

- In 31 March 2003, 157,000 people were on the register of blind people, a decrease of 1100 (almost 1%) since March 2000.
- 13,000 people joined the register of blind people during 2002–2003, about the same number of people joining as in 1999–2000.
- In 31 March 2003, 155,000 people were on the register of partially sighted people, an increase of 6500 (about 4%) since March 2000.
- 16,600 people joined the register of partially sighted people during 2002–2003, about 900 fewer people than in 1999–2000.
- 25% of all registered blind people who had an additional disability were also recorded as deaf or having a hearing impairment.
- 23% of all registered partially sighted people who had an additional disability were also deaf or had a hearing impairment.

Scotland[20]

Main findings

- In 2003, the number of people registered as blind or partially sighted was estimated to be 38,000, up 2% on 2002.
- There were 3491 new cases registered during the period 1 April 2002 to 31 March 2003. This was down by 7% on 2002.
- The majority, 62%, of those on the register were blind, and 38% were partially sighted.
- 36% of those on the register were male and 64% were female.
- Almost four out of five of those registered were over the age of 65.
- 7693 persons (20%) of those registered as visually impaired had additional disabilities. Of these, 35% were deaf.

Table 2.2 Registered blind and partially sighted people: year ending 31 March 2003, England[22]

England 2003	Total number of people registered	Age 0 to 4	Age 5 to 17	Age 18 to 49	Age 50 to 64	Age 65 to 74	Age 75 or over
Registered blind	156,680	725	3230	17,090	14,520	15,460	105,655
Registered partially sighted	155,230	585	4230	15,315	12,935	16,640	105,525

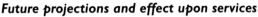

Future projections and effect upon services

More recently there has become a greater need and emphasis on retaining independence within the community and therefore it follows that there will be a greater number of visually impaired patients within the community who require services and an improved access to advice, assistance and information.

There are also many who are not registered at all, and even more who fall below hospital referral criteria, but who still have a degree of visual impairment. Many of them are patients who attend regular eye examinations within our busy practices.

Common causes

Children

It is unusual to have a child attend for an eye examination within the General Ophthalmic Service with a previously unrecognized or unreported condition. Most congenital conditions are apparent from an early age and these children tend to be seen within the Hospital Eye Service until early adulthood, even if the condition is non-progressive.

Accurate statistics of visual impairment in children are hard to obtain, as it is not necessary for children to be registered. However, it is understood that the most common cause of visual disability in children is optic atrophy, whether this has been caused by some perinatal event or whether it has been inherited.

Most common causes in children
- Optic atrophy.
- Congenital cataract.
- Congenital idiopathic nystagmus.
- Congenital abnormalities of the brain and nervous system.

Early adult life
- Stargardt's disease.
- Retinitis pigmentosa.

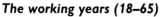
The working years (18–65)
- Diabetic retinopathy: most common cause.
- Myopia.
- Uveitis.
- Corneal dystrophies.
- Degenerative conditions such as cataract and macular disease are significantly present.

In retirement
- Cataracts are the largest single cause of visual impairment, but in most cases vision may be restored by surgery.
- Age-related macular degeneration: greatest cause of irreversible visual impairment diabetic retinopathy.
- Glaucoma.
- Retinal detachments.

Age-related macular degeneration
Thanks to an improvement in recent years of systemic conditions such as diabetes and heart disease, people are living for longer and the prevalence of degenerative conditions such as ARMD is increasing. Although far from complete, the projections accurately depict that the majority of our visually impaired patients are elderly. Evans in 1995[19] found that 90% of people with a serious sight problem were over 60 years of age. Shaw[23] suggested that this figure would increase by almost 30% in the next 20 years. Owen et al.[18] concluded that although the estimates of visual impairment caused by ARMD were well below other figures often cited, the results pooled from six studies showed that the prevalence of visual loss caused by ARMD increased exponentially from the age of 70–85 years, with 3.5% having visual impairment beyond the age of 75 years. The authors estimate that there are currently 214,000 with visual impairment caused by ARMD (suitable for registration) and this number is expected to increase to 239,000 by the year 2011.

The Department of Health has estimated that the total number of visually impaired is set to rise by 25% in the next 20 years.[2] This will undoubtedly have the effect of a greater demand for services for visually impaired people, which will include the provision of low vision aids.

3
Adapting the eye examination for the visually impaired

3
Adapting the eye examination for the visually impaired

Consulting room equipment

Despite the significant number of visually impaired people within the community, many consulting rooms are poorly equipped to see patients with even a mild degree of visual impairment.

Below is a guide to useful consulting room equipment and alterations that can be made to permit an easier examination of our visually impaired patients.

Distance acuity test charts

Snellen acuity test cards[24]

Snellen acuity test cards (Fig. 3.1) are argued to have limited value when testing visually impaired patients.[25,26] This is mainly because:

- There are too few letters below 6/18 and only one single 6/60 sized letter which may or may not be seen, depending on the location and size of a central scotoma, corneal scar or cataract.
- There is an inconsistency in letter legibility. Some of the letters are easier to identify than others. With fewer choices of letters at the lower acuity levels, this will have an impact on overall accuracy.
- There is an inconsistent size ratio between consecutive lines. For example, 6/60 is 1.67 times larger than 6/24, but 6/6 is 1.2 times larger than 6/5.
- The spacing between rows and between letters is again inconsistent and bears no relationship between the height and width of the letters. Therefore, when the chart is used at a closer working distance than 6 m, the patient will read further down the chart and therefore have additional bearing on the accuracy of the measurement of V/VA.[26]

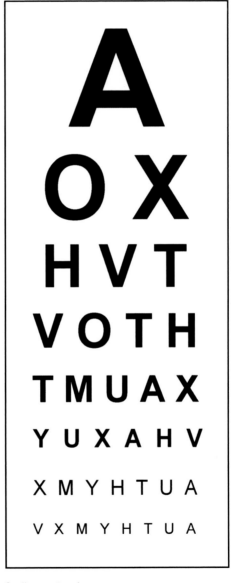

Figure 3.1 Snellen acuity chart

- With the spacing between letters inconsistent, the lower lines of letters are more crowded. Therefore the 6/12 line at 1 meter is not an equivalent target to 6/24 at 2 meters.

Despite the limitations of Snellen acuity cards being well known, they continue to persist as the most commonly used measurement of spatial vision, as a result of being very sensitive to refractive error and blur.

Bailey–Lovie logMAR acuity charts

The advantages of **logMAR** acuity and the development of the Bailey–Lovie charts have been well documented.[25,27–32] In summary:

- Line and letter spacing equivalent throughout the chart (Fig. 3.2). The spacing between each letter and each row is related to the width and height of the letters, respectively.
- Consistent size ratio. The magnification is the same between successive lines, 1.25× (or 0.1 log units).
- All letters are chosen for equal legibility.
- There is an equal number of letters on each line, typically five on a Bailey–Lovie chart.
- The final logMAR score takes into consideration all letters that have been read successfully.

Visually impaired patients are now able to read from a choice of five letters on each line. This is often found to be more encouraging, especially for those patients who have been previously familiar with just one or two letters, at the top of a Snellen chart. The chart is easily converted for use at different distances, and is therefore useful for refracting patients with acuities below 6/60, and is furthermore encouraging for those patients who have not been able to see a chart at all in previous examinations. Just as there are matching single letter versions of the Snellen chart (such as the Sheridan–Gardiner cards), there are matching line targets (such as the Sonksen–Silver cards), useful for those patients unfamiliar with or unable to read out letters.

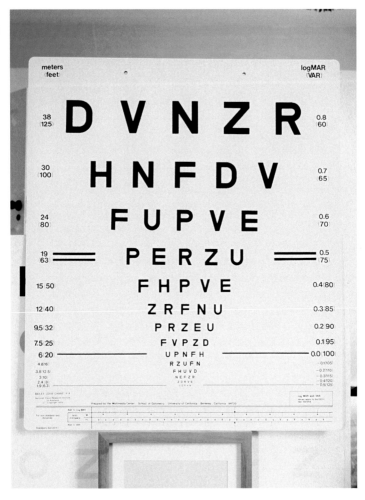

Figure 3.2 logMAR acuity chart

Test Chart 2000 and 2000^{PRO}

The potential of computer monitors for the display of visual test stimuli is well recognized.[33] It is possible to achieve high contrast, to display information with uniform illumination and they are highly adaptable to achieve variation of color, contrast and spatial configurations.

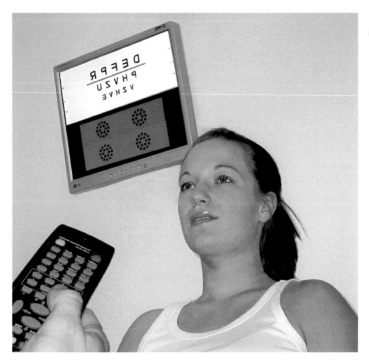

Figure 3.3 Test Chart 2000

The Test Chart 2000 and 2000^PRO (Fig. 3.3) can be run on any PC or laptop that supports Microsoft Windows, providing a versatile and cost-effective alternative to conventional back-illuminated or projection charts. It has rapidly become an ideal option in test chart equipment, offering a full range of tests. It is also extremely useful for domiciliary work as the chart can be reconfigured for any working distance and be run direct from a laptop computer.

Vision/visual acuity (V/VA) measurements can be taken using Snellen, logMAR and Sloan notations with the additional advantage of testing at low contrasts. Furthermore, there is also included a Pelli–Robson Low Contrast Letter Chart which has been well documented to be of use in assessing a patient's visual performance in real-world situations.[25,34–36]

Near vision charts

The Faculty of Ophthalmologists Times New Roman near chart

The Faculty of Ophthalmologists Times New Roman chart for near vision is still the most widely used in optometric practice. It offers high contrast blocks of text ranging from N48 to N5 or in some cases N4.5. The relationship of print size is easily understood. N5 is half the size of N10; N18 is three times larger than N6, etc. While an accurate measurement of near acuity is arguably required for comparisons between successive visits, many patients comment that the high contrast of the printed test card (≥90%) bears less resemblance to the ability to read at home. Most newsprint and paperback novels are printed in lower contrast (75% approx), which may become further reduced with age and use. There is also the risk of glare when the card is laminated.

Reading is a complex task and beyond the scope of this book. Measurement of reading with the Times New Roman chart is not the smallest size of letter that can be resolved. It is the ability to read words and blocks of test that are being tested and not single letters, as on a distance acuity test. There is meaning within the blocks of text that will help a patient in being able to read a whole word and follow a passage of meaningful text.

Bailey–Lovie word reading chart

The near Bailey–Lovie chart has all the advantages of a logarithmic scale. It tests from N80 to N2 with a random selection of words, allowing improved testing of threshold near acuity. This furthermore becomes advantageous when testing reading performance with low vision devices, where improved fluency is determined by allowing a certain amount of acuity 'in reserve'. It is, therefore, useful to have a chart displaying print of a size several steps smaller than the target print size a patient may wish to achieve. However, at the larger sizes there are a limited number of words available and, therefore, it is unfeasible to assess the quality of a patient's reading performance with this chart.

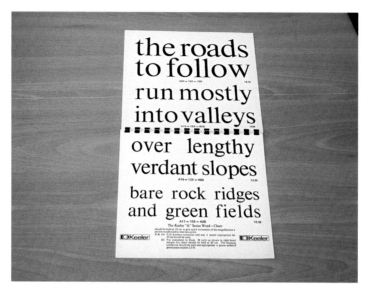

Figure 3.4   Keeler A series chart

Keeler A series chart

The Keeler A series chart (Fig. 3.4) has a logarithmic progression.

In the Keeler A system the letter size labeled as A1 has lower case letters whose overall angular subtense at the test's designated standard distance of 25 cm is 5′ of arc (Table 3.1).

The A system was originally designed to aid the practitioner in calculating the magnification required for low vision devices. However, one significant disadvantage of the system is that the word separation does not bear resemblance to normal printed text. Based on a working distance of 25 cm, with the patient appropriately corrected, Table 3.2 gives the magnification required to improve the vision to a different level.

MNREAD acuity charts (Figs. 3.5a,b)

The Minnesota Low-Vision Reading Test is a computer-based system for measuring reading speed.[37] This test has more recently

Table 3.1 **Comparison of Times New Roman and Keeler 'A' Series fonts**

Times New Roman	Keeler 'A' Series
	A1
	A2
	A3
	A4
N5	A5
N6	A6
N8	A7 Newsprint
N10	A8
N12	A9
N18	A11
	A12
N24	A13
N36	A14
N48	
	A17

been created as a printed card version for use within clinical practice.[37,38] The cards are printed in high contrast, including reverse contrast, and print size varies from logMAR 1.3 to −0.5 (N64 to N1). The practitioner records the time taken for the patient to read a sentence of unrelated words, each of the same length (60 characters, 10 standard length words), and reads down the charts until mistakes are made. The cards have been demonstrated to have significant value on the evaluation of reading performance and are becoming more widely used in low vision clinics.[25,34,37–43]

Table 3.2 **Magnification relationship for Keeler 'A' Series print sizes**

Visual acuity	Magnification required to raise visual acuity to					
'A' Series	A10	A9	A8	A7	A6	A5
A6						1.3
A7					1.3	1.6
A8				1.3	1.6	2
A9			1.3	1.6	2	2.5
A10		1.3	1.6	2	2.5	3
A11	1.3	1.6	2	2.5	3	4
A12	1.6	2	2.5	3	4	5
A13	2	2.5	3	4	5	6
A14	2.5	3	4	5	6	8
A15	3	4	5	6	8	10
A16	4	5	6	8	10	12
A17	5	6	8	10	12	15
A18	6	8	10	12	15	18
A19	8	10	12	15	18	23
A20	10	12	15	18	23	

The McClure Reading Test (Fig. 3.6)

The McClure Reading Test has been designed specifically for use with children. It contains reading material of varying difficulty or standards, appropriate for different age groups. It is important to be able to assess the child's ability to see to read rather than their ability to read, especially for those children who have difficulty reading aloud. However, one disadvantage is that the

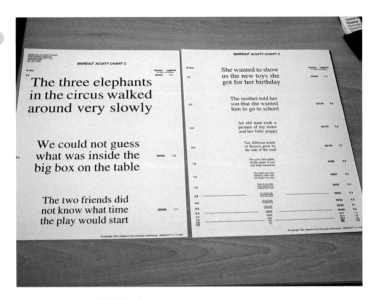

Figure 3.5a MNREAD chart

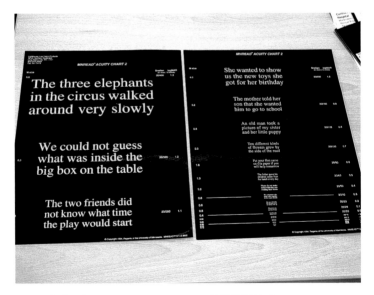

Figure 3.5b Reverse contrast version of MNREAD chart

CHILDRENS READING TYPE
age group 4-5 years

N5
the cat has a toy
here is a pig
the pig can run
the red rug can the shop
I can see the rug
the boy can see the pig the toy pig is in the shop

N6
here is a ball
the girl likes the ball
the ball is in the big tree
the cat likes to play with the toy and the ball the toy is big

N8
here is a toy
the boy plays with the toy
the toy is on the red rug
the cat likes the rug
the cat plays with the boy on the rug
the boy likes to play with the cat

N10
here is a tree
the tree is wet
the ball is in the tree
I like the girl
the girl runs to the tree for the ball
the ball is big and wet

N12
here is a cat
the cat has a toy
the boy plays with the cat
the cat likes the toy
the girl and the boy play with the cat
the dog can run with the boy

N14
here is a dog
the dog can run
the girl likes the dog
the girl has fun
the dog can run for the ball
the girl and the dog have fun

age group 5-6 years

N5
Here is a dog and here is a ball
The dog has fun with the ball
I can see the dog in the shop
I like the sweets in the shop
The dog plays with the toy and ball. I can get the ball

N6
Here is a girl and here is a cat
The girl can play with the cat and a toy
They play by the big tree
They have fun with that toy
The cat can run to get the toy. The girl has fun with the cat

N8
Here is a boy and here is a big dog
They have fun with the ball
The ball is in the water and the
dog jumps into the water
The dog can get the ball from the water,
but the boy can not get the fish.

N10
Here is a pig and here is a tree
I can see the pig and the big tree
I like to play with a ball and have fun
Here is some water by the tree
The pig can go to the water.
He can see a big fish in the water.

N12
Here is a girl and here is a shop
It is a sweet shop and a toy shop
The girl likes the toys in the shop
She can have fun with the toys
The girl can go to the shop to get some dolls
She can get big toys in the shop

N14
Here is a man and here is a cat
The cat has fun with a toy
They are on the red rug
The cat can sit with the man.
We like to see the cat have fun.
The man has to go home to see the cat.

Figure 3.6 Samples from the McClure Reading Test showing print for different age groups (Reproduced with permission from Harvey & Gilmartin, *Paediatric Optometry*, Butterworth-Heinemann)

child's age group appears at the top of the printed text, and this can be off-putting for those children who are sensitive to their reading capabilities. [For a full description of targets useful for visually impaired children, see Harper, R. (2004) *Low-Vision Assessment and Management* in Harvey & Gilmartin, *Paediatric Optometry*, Butterworth-Heinemann.]

Alternative reading materials
Once accurate measurement of acuity and reading performance have been made, it can be useful to have a selection of everyday print available for the patient to use when assessing the usefulness of low vision devices. For example, it may be necessary to obtain a selection of print in other languages. Magazines and newspapers are also important, as are catalogs, maps and photographs, particularly for children. Books, including large print books and bibles, are also useful. It is also possible to acquire public examination papers, in normal and large print.

Other refraction equipment

Basic refraction equipment is all that is necessary to examine visually impaired patients. A suitable trial frame is preferred to a phoropter head. The latter tends to obstruct patients who would probably adopt an abnormal head posture. Such patients would include those with a central scotoma who prefer to adopt an eccentric view for testing distance acuity, and similarly, those with nystagmus. A Halberg clip is also useful for those patients, as they may prefer to keep their current correction in place in order to adopt their usual head posture. The phoropter also has the disadvantage of reducing the light levels that may influence a person's visual capability. It also prevents the practitioner from observing patient facial expression, something of great use to the experienced practitioner.

In addition to the usual equipment for refraction, cross-cylinder lenses of ±0.75, ±1.00 and $\pm1.50DC$ are available. The first two are the most useful as the ±1.50 gives a presentation difference of 3D, which is often deemed too large even for those with a poor acuity. Binocular twirls are also available in similar powers.

±0.25 sphere and cyl changes have limited value on any low vision patient with acuity of less than 6/24. It is important to remember that, even with lower levels of impairment, the ability to discriminate between two blurred presentations fall dramatically. Added to this, in a central scotoma, acuity may often be very variable during a subjective routine. The need for accuracy must always be balanced with a realistic view about the patient's subjective response reliability.

Low vision kits and devices

There are a number of comprehensive low vision assessment sets available. A full list of major UK suppliers is given in the appendices. The practitioner is advised to have a good look around before purchasing large expensive devices.

Many concentrate on spectacle magnifiers and spectacle mounted telescopes for near and distance. While these are important to have for low vision assessments, it must be remembered that by far the majority of low vision devices prescribed to the elderly are usually simple hand and stand magnifiers.

The first visit

Like any other eye examination, it is important to follow a well-constructed and methodical routine. The first thing to determine is what it is that the patient wants to be able to do (within reason), and then take appropriate action to meet those needs. This may include prescribing magnification, giving advice on lighting or eccentric viewing strategies, or perhaps discussing further referral onto social services for rehabilitation and training.

The practitioner needs to take a positive approach and modify the consultation accordingly. We need to listen to what the patient has to say. The objective is not to prescribe something that fits, but it is to take an approach that this could be the first in a number of consultations. Frustrations expressed by the practitioner will have a negative effect on the patient and there will be less likelihood of success. A low vision aid is not the 'end of the road', but an enhancement of the new or recent situation. References to how life used to be needs to be discussed with care, as are references to what it could have been, for those with a congenital loss.

Real benefit may be gained from a thorough discussion with the patient. Often patients have uncertain or erroneous knowledge about their eye condition and a clear explanation and reassurance is often as valuable as a magnifier. A good example of this is when an elderly patient has developed neovascular macular degeneration in a short period of time. This is a difficult disease process for many undergraduates to fully comprehend and when compounded by central vision loss and a lack of medical help, the main obstacle to the patient adapting to their new visual environment is often one of understanding.

Table 3.3 **A useful guide for assessing low vision patients**

Guide to initial consultation

1. History and symptoms

   a. Determine the patient's lifestyle, daily living requirements, work or education requirements and special hobbies.

   b. Determine the disease process and the patient's understanding of it, previous or pending treatments and whether the condition has stabilized.

   c. Determine previous registration, and social service communications.

   d. Discuss the usefulness and/or limitations of any current aids in use.

   e. Discuss the problems encountered with any previously used devices.

2. A detailed task analysis

   a. Size and working distance.

   b. Spot checks or fluency?

3. Current spectacles and LVAs (low vision aids) in use

4. Assessment of visual function

   a. Determine current refraction: modifications needed.

   b. Determine or calculate the degree of magnification required to meet specific tasks previously identified.

   c. Identify an appropriate aid to meet the required task, where appropriate.

5. Prescribing and follow up

   a. Determine whether the patient requires further assistance from other professionals and give appropriate advice and information.

   b. Follow up as required.

Determining the magnification and the most appropriate aid for the desired task must be approached systematically yet with a flexible attitude (Table 3.3). Consulting time will then be dramatically reduced and confidence restored.

Before the assessment

Many practitioners feel that an initial questionnaire, sent to the patient, is useful in helping the patient to focus on their individual problem prior to the consultation.

Wolffsohn and Cochrane designed a questionnaire called the Low Vision Quality of Life Questionnaire (LVQOL)[44] (Table 3.4) which has been successfully implemented by post.[45] It is available in large print.

If available, a report from a rehabilitation worker is very useful. This is increasingly the case where a clinic has been set up in liaison with local social services and, as dedicated local schemes become more the norm, such interprofessional integration will greatly improve the effectiveness of the help on offer to the visually impaired.

History and symptoms

> **Determine the patient's lifestyle, daily living requirements and special hobbies**

The following section will deal with the examination and low vision assessment with particular reference to an elderly patient. All such information gathering should be tailored to the patient's individual circumstance and so will vary. For example, in the case of a visually impaired child, many of the points described in Chapter 10 regarding statementing, educational resource, and so on, will also need to be ascertained.

Table 3.4 The Low Vision Quality-of-Life Questionnaire (LVQOL)

Distance Vision, Mobility and Lighting	Grading					
How much of a problem do you have:	None	Moderate		Great		
With your vision in general	5	4	3	2	1	x	n/a
With your eyes getting tired (e.g. only being able to do a task for a short time)	5	4	3	2	1	x	n/a
With your vision at night inside the house	5	4	3	2	1	x	n/a
Getting the right amount of light to be able to see	5	4	3	2	1	x	n/a
With glare (e.g. dazzled by car lights or the sun)	5	4	3	2	1	x	n/a
Seeing street signs	5	4	3	2	1	x	n/a
Seeing the television (appreciating the pictures)	5	4	3	2	1	x	n/a
Seeing moving objects (e.g. cars on the road)	5	4	3	2	1	x	n/a
With judging the depth or distance of items (e.g. reaching for a glass)	5	4	3	2	1	x	n/a
Seeing steps or curbs	5	4	3	2	1	x	n/a

Getting around outdoors (e.g. on uneven pavements) because of your vision	5	4	3	2	1	x	n/a
Crossing a road with traffic because of your vision	5	4	3	2	1	x	n/a

Adjustment

Because of your vision, are you:	**No**		**Moderately**		**Greatly**		
Unhappy at your situation in life	5	4	3	2	1	x	n/a
Frustrated at not being able to do certain tasks	5	4	3	2	1	x	n/a
Restricted in visiting friends or family	5	4	3	2	1	x	n/a
	Well				**Poorly**	**Not explained**	
How well has your eye condition been explained to you	5	4	3	2	1	x	

Reading and Fine Work

With your reading aids/glasses, if used, how much of a problem do you have:	**None**		**Moderate**		**Great**		
Reading large print (e.g. newspaper headlines)	5	4	3	2	1	x	n/a
Reading newspaper text and books	5	4	3	2	1	x	n/a

Continued

Table 3.4 The Low Vision Quality-of-Life Questionnaire (LVQOL)—cont'd

	None		Moderate		Great		
Reading labels (e.g. on medicine bottles)	5	4	3	2	1	x	n/a
Reading your letters and mail	5	4	3	2	1	x	n/a
Having problems using tools (e.g. threading a needle or cutting)	5	4	3	2	1	x	n/a

Activities of Daily Living

With your reading aids/glasses, if used, how much of a problem do you have:	None		Moderate		Great		
Finding out the time for yourself	5	4	3	2	1	x	n/a
Writing (e.g. check or cards)	5	4	3	2	1	x	n/a
Reading your own handwriting	5	4	3	2	1	x	n/a
With your everyday activities (e.g. household chores)	5	4	3	2	1	x	n/a

Reprinted from The American Journal of Ophthalmology, Vol: 130, Wolffsohn and Cochrane, Design of the low vision quality of life questionnaire (LVQOL) and measuring the outcome of low vision rehabilitation, pages 793–802, Copyright (2000), with permission

Initiating the discussion

'How do you think I can help you today?'

A broad opening question of this nature gives the patient the opportunity to reveal to what extent he is aware of the service you can offer him. It is important to be aware of his expectations as this may have some bearing on his motivation. It is not uncommon to have patients who have been told a variety of misinformation, which can often be a large initial hurdle to overcome.

For example, is he aware of the service that you are able to offer him, or has he been told that he can be offered 'stronger glasses'?

During the opening remarks it is often very valuable for the practitioners to introduce themselves and explain their role. Bear in mind that the patient may well have seen several eye care professionals by the time they reach the optometrist and may be somewhat confused about what might be achieved. An initial introduction not only allows the practitioner to help the patient relax, but also may limit any unrealistic expectations the patient may have about the outcome of the assessment from the outset.

'I am going to ask a few questions about your eyes and the sorts of things you need to be able to see. I will then measure the vision you have and find out if there is any way we can help you to use it'.

Notice how this approach avoids words such as 'improve' or 'make better' which may come back to haunt the practitioner.

Level of vision and the effect on lifestyle

'Can you describe to me what sort of problems you have been having since your vision deteriorated?
How has the visual impairment affected your day-to-day situation?'

A loss of visual function will have brought about significant lifestyle changes. By establishing these from the start, the practitioner can begin to address individual needs.

Therefore, build a picture of the patient's everyday life, and make a note to return to specific points when performing a detailed task analysis. For example:

- Unable to drive
- Unable to read personal mail
- Unable to see VDU
- Unable to see blackboard
- Unable to see train indicator boards

A sample selection of questions:

What size of print would you like to be able to see?
What size of print do you need to be able to see?
What size of print are you managing to see at the moment?
Are you able to read and reply to your own mail?
Are you having difficulty with the cooker dials/washing machine, etc.?
Do you live alone?
Do you have extra help? From whom?
Are you mobile? Are you able to get out on your own?

Do you need to cook for yourself?
Are you able to go shopping alone for food?
For other essential items?
Are you able to see the prices in the supermarket?
Are you able to guide yourself about the aisles?
Are you aware that you can ask for assistance if you are visually impaired?
How do you get there?

How do you occupy the day?

Once the list is made of individual tasks, it is then important to discuss the significance of each and determine whether the patient is handicapped by the loss of function. For example, the inability to see a train indicator board may not hold any significance to the patient if he has no plans of using public transport on a regular basis. However, some patients may have stopped using public transport because they are no longer confident in doing so, rather than the fact that they have no special need to. On the other hand, the inability to see the VDU will have obvious employment significance if the patient's job depends on it.

Practitioners should make themselves aware of whether the patient has a need for independence and whether the patient lives alone or not. If they have become isolated, is this a consequence of their condition or as a result of poor advice and information, or perhaps other factors, such as poor English or other cultural factors? In the same respect, the patient's mobility is also worthy of further questioning. Do they have a need for getting out more? Is it their sight that is restricting them from going out more or is it to do with another medical problem?

Are there any other medical problems that may have a bearing on mobility, or how they may use any device? Do they have additional help in the home? Do they have supportive friends, neighbors or relatives close by?

Many elderly patients live alone and may have other disabilities. However, it is better not to make assumptions. Each individual is treated equally, taking their age into consideration for some practicalities, but leave many questions open. Individuals will respond to their situation in different ways. Having a partner, spouse or parent at home can make a significant difference in their lifestyle and the ability to cope with the situation.

> **Determine the disease process. Previous or pending treatments and whether it has stabilized**

Can you tell me what you know about your condition?
How long has this been affecting you?
For how long has your vision been at this level?
Has it changed recently?
Can you tell me what treatment you have already had?
Do you have any further hospital appointments?
Do you have any pending treatment?
When is your next appointment?
With whom?
Have you been discharged?

Many patients, despite having been through the hospital system, may still have a poor appreciation of their condition. It is important for the practitioner to have an understanding of how they perceive the impairment, as this will reflect upon the motivation to use devices. After all, if a patient believes that pending treatment will reverse rather than stop the progression of the disease process, they may not be willing to use a device. Macular degeneration is particularly difficult for many patients to understand and the role of the optometrist in explaining is very important; arguably one of the main ways they can help.

Determine previous registration and social service communications

---

Have you been certified severely sight impaired/blind or sight impaired/partially sighted?
For how long?
Have you been registered with the local Primary Care Trust?
When did this happen?
Have you had a visit from Social Services yet?
What did they do for you?
Did you find the advice/information/equipment useful?
Do you feel that you need to speak to someone again?
Do you feel that your vision has become worse since your first certification?
Do you feel that you have received good advice or do you have questions left unanswered?
Have you moved since your registration and if so, have you been re-registered?

Other aids, e.g. the Talking Book Service?
Enlarged bank statement?
Do they go to a blind society?

Most patients are not aware that Social Services accept self-referrals. Under Community Care Legislation[46] a patient is entitled to a home visit and assistance from Social Services if they demonstrate the 'need'. If they have already been added to the Primary Care Trust's register of blind and partially sighted, then a phone call should be the only thing that separates them from another visit from a member of staff.

Examples of some regular observations made by patients which may warrant individual consideration:

---

1. Effect of lighting: *contrast sensitivity.*

2. Glare sources: *contrast sensitivity.*
3. Coping strategies: *psychological adaptability.*
4. Face recognition: *central scotomas.*
5. Problems with mobility: *visual fields.*

A detailed task analysis

- **Size and working distance of the task/s?**
- **Spot checks or fluency?**

Size and working distance of the task

There is the need to be specific. It is usual to have a variety of print qualities and sizes in the consulting room, for example, newspapers, magazines or catalogs, large print books and bibles. It is often a good idea for the patient to bring a sample of the print that they need to be able to see with them, including textbooks, etc., for children and students.

Examples, which may indicate the use of a near device:

- Shop prices.
- Packets in the supermarket.
- Newsprint, novels.
- Large print books (standard print N10–12, large print N18–24).
- Coins and banknotes.
- Post/letters/TV listings.
- Knitting patterns.
- Signing cheques.
- Dialing the telephone.
- Bank statements.

Distance examples, which may indicate mobility training, or the use of a distance device:

- Mobility, crossing the road.
- Watching television.
- Watching football, cricket, etc., at the grounds.
- Traveling on the underground.
- Train indicator boards.

Spot checks or fluent reading?

The task will dictate either spot or fluent reading. This will have a bearing on the strength of magnification prescribed and the type of device issued. For example, a patient who needs a device such as a hand magnifier to check the cooker dials will require different magnification and possibly a separate type of device for reading his large print book, even if the size of the task is the same. For fluent reading a certain amount of **acuity reserve** may be required as working near the threshold will be too difficult for the patient and the outcome likely to be less successful.[25,34] Where a patient has complained of glare or difficulties with varying light levels, very often a deficit in contrast sensitivity is measurable and in this case a **contrast reserve** needs to be considered when prescribing.

General health

Other aspects of a typical examination will still need to be taken into consideration for the usual reasons. Detail may be sought regarding a general medical condition when it has a bearing on the use of a low vision device. For example, a patient whose hands are severely arthritic may have difficulty in using a hand-held device. The visual impairment may be to the detriment of their general medical condition, for example, when a patient has difficulties in distinguishing the various medications they have been prescribed for their heart condition. This may often only be discovered after specific questioning.

In summary

The above lists are by no means exhaustive. The practitioner will guide, and be guided by, the needs of the individual. The patient will remember more as the consultation proceeds, in particular will have more to say when they themselves have a clearer indication regarding what you can do. A friend or family member may additionally aid the process if they are allowed to sit in on the consultation.

However, it is important to set out expectations from the start. All devices will be a compromise to an individual who has previously had 'normal sight', and the use of these will be determined by the way in which the practitioner manages the consultation, degree of motivation behind the patient, and, ultimately, the patient's level of visual acuity.

Build up a picture of the patient's needs, expectations and motivation

---

- Are they actually interested in reading again?
- Have they given up or will they try? Sadly, too many visually impaired suffer in silence, often alone, under the misconception that there is nothing that can be done and that visual tasks are no longer available to them.
- If they say that they are not reading is it because they are not interested or is it because they cannot see well enough?
- Do not subscribe to stereotypes (many very elderly still wish to surf the internet, for example, so do not limit questions about expectations to assumed stereotypical age behavior).

Current spectacles and LVAs in use

- Discuss the usefulness and/or limitations of any current aids in use.
- Discuss the problems encountered with previously used devices.

---

1. Have you tried using a magnifier?
2. Where/from whom did you get it?
3. Did you find it useful?
4. What can you manage to do with it?
5. What could you not manage with it?

> ### Case example 1   Mr T
>
> #### History and symptoms
>
> Age 75, lives with disabled wife. No longer driving (3 years). Retired. ARMD diagnosed 5 years ago. No hospital treatment, discharged from main clinic. Was seen once in low vision clinic 4 years ago, given hand magnifier for newspaper. Did not feel the need for follow up. Managed well, until recently. Used now for large print only, feels vision has deteriorated in past few months.
>
> Registered PS 5 years ago. Has Talking Books and home help 4 days to help with disabled wife (normal sight, wheelchair bound). Has not felt the need to contact social services since initial visit following registration 5 years ago.
>
> Managing own personal finances and correspondence fairly well with current hand magnifier, but would like to read novels (is not happy with the list of large print books from library) but says would settle with the newspaper for now.
>
> Keen follower of local and national cricket, has problems seeing scoreboard. Managing to cook, has put large stickers on dials, etc., in kitchen. Occasional problems with cooking instructions when home help away.
>
> Manages buses fine. Son lives local, although rarely seen.
>
> Motivation good.

6. Has your vision worsened since you were prescribed/bought the device?

7. Can you show me how you use it?

8. Do you use it with or without your spectacles?

9. If it were taken away, would you miss it?

It is essential for the patient to bring all current spectacles and low vision aids to the consulting room whether they are in use or not. If the patient has had a visual impairment for some time, then it is likely that they will have already tried using a magnifier. Even if it is one they used for stamp collecting 20 years ago, discuss its limitations: 'what can they or can they not do with it?'

> ### *Case example 2* **Mrs M**
>
> Daughter also in attendance today.
>
> ### History and symptoms
>
> Age 72. Widow. Lives alone. Daughter, husband and three teenage grandsons live next door. Retired, not driving. Active within the church and Women's Institute.
>
> Diabetic. Left eye (LE) blind due to retinal detachment 10 years ago. Feels this was caused by an unsuccessful cataract operation. Macular hole (right eye, RE) for 5 years. No treatment. Aware of advancing cataract RE. Not keen on treatment. Attends eye hospital yearly for check. Last visit 2 months ago. Outcome stable. Not registered blind or partially sighted. Does not appear aware of help available from social services.
>
> Has not been prescribed any low vision aids. Has tried using own hand magnifier to read cookery books and TV listings but prefers to remove own spectacles instead. Is only able to manage headlines of a newspaper for the last year.
>
> Dependent on daughter to read own mail but would like to be able to read knitting patterns, wine and cookery books and look at personal photographs. Says not interested in novels or talking books, as she hasn't the time.
>
> Hobbies include hill walking, cookery and wine tasting.
>
> Motivation fair.

Ask them to bring it along with them to the examination. Often, by simply increasing the addition in their current spectacles may mean that they can use the aid they already have more efficiently. Also, it is not uncommon to find that a patient has been using the wrong spectacles with a stand magnifier.

It is a useful exercise to go through each device or pair of spectacles in the consulting room; the practitioner may also pick up more information about managing expectations and the degree of patient motivation.

Record type, approximate age, condition and equivalent lens power of magnifier

- A full description necessary for easy identification.
- Record specifically what each aid is used for, its shortfalls, level of vision achieved and the working distance, if relevant.

The magnification of hand and stand magnifiers can be noted in two ways, the trade magnification and nominal magnification formulae. The former formula refers to the magnification of hand and stand magnifiers. Thus, if we are to be certain about the exact power of the device, it is always advisable to note the equivalent lens power as well. This avoids confusion between practitioners during successive visits.

Example

A ×6 stand magnifier could indicate either a +20D or +24D lens, depending on which formula the manufacturer has used.

Trade magnification formula	**Nominal magnification formula**
$M = F/4+1$	$M = F/4$
$6 = F/4+1$	$6 = F/4$
$F = 20D$	$F = 24D$

Mr T

Bifocals 5 years old, condition—scratched.

R	**L**
$+2.75/-0.75 \times 180 = 6/24^{+1}$	$+3.50/-1.25 \times 175 = 6/60$
logMAR 0.58	logMAR 1.00
Add +2.75 = N12 at 30 cm	Add +2.75 = N24 at 32 cm

In use

Coil Windsor Hand magnifier (very scratched) +7.00D.
Achieves N10 fair (R eye); handling good.
Complains 'not enough light'.

- Mr T may be happy with using a hand magnifier, but one that is in poor condition will give a poor quality image. One would expect a +7.00D magnifier to improve his near visual acuity better than to N10.
- It may also be necessary to consider an illuminated version while reviewing the strength. N10 may be useful for his day-to-day correspondence, but it will not be enough to be able to manage sustained reading as it is too near threshold acuity.

Mrs M

Bifocals 2 years old, from HES, good condition:

R	L
$-2.75/-2.50 \times 165$ = 3/36	-3.50 Balance = NPL (no
logMAR 1.06	perception of light)

Add +3.50   = N24 at 40 cm

Unaided NV: N18 at 20 cm

Brought but no longer used

Own hand magnifier (scratched[+]) +10.00D

Tends to use without any spectacles: achieves N24 well, but handling very poor.

- Mrs M explained that she had been given a stronger reading segment by the hospital 2 years ago, but had been unable to get used to it. As a result, she was not keen to have 'stronger glasses' again.
- It also appeared that the working distance of her +3.50 addition was 40 cm. A 40 cm working distance would normally equate to an addition of +2.50. As the print blurred closer than this 40 cm working distance, it would suggest that there had been a recent myopic shift in her distance prescription. (A +3.50 addition would have a working distance of 100/3.5 = 28 cm.) This is further supported by an unaided near vision of N18 at a working distance of -5D.

Assessment of visual function

Visually impaired patients often find visual assessment stressful and occasionally distressing, especially when they are aware of a drop in vision or another reduction in visual function. It is not uncommon for the patient to be anxious and, therefore, it is worth taking the time to make him or her comfortable and to leave as much time as possible. A patient who is stressed may not perform as well as they can and, therefore, the accuracy of the assessment could be compromised.

It is worth investing in a test chart that can test low visual acuities quickly and efficiently. The single 6/60 letter on a standard Snellen 6/60 chart will not be sufficient for accuracy or repeatability. It also reinforces the impairment to the patient at a time when it is important to be encouraging.

Recording distance vision/visual acuities

It is essential to be as accurate as possible. A small drop in visual acuity due to poor repeatability can easily be misinterpreted as a further loss due to ongoing pathology. Secondly, the relationship between distance and near acuities and subsequent magnification calculations will be much easier if there is an accurate starting point. For example, don't use counting fingers or <6/6/0. Neither will give a repeatable or useful measurement.

If a standard Snellen chart is all that is available, move it closer and give the patient the option of looking at more letters. However, be aware of the impact this will have on the acuity measurement, and, therefore, record the distance at which the chart is moved to, to ensure accuracy between successive visits.

For a logMAR chart, do not forget that less good acuity is noted as a higher number. Every letter on a line is given a value of 0.02. So if a patient reads every letter but one on the 0.9 line of a 4 meter logMAR chart at 4 meters then acuity is recorded as 0.92. If they read all of the line and one letter on the following line, then the score is 0.88.

For logMAR charts, a useful rule of thumb is to add 0.3 for every time the distance of the chart is halved. So if at 4 meters the patient fails to read the letters but at 2 meters manages four of the top five letters, then this would be scored as 1.32 (1.0 score at 4 meters plus 0.02 for the missing letter and plus 0.3 for the halved working distance).

When using line targets, it is also useful to note whether the patient is using eccentric viewing to see the letters. If they can only see the end letters when looking at the central letter, a note might be made of this as this patient may well benefit from encouragement to exploit this eccentric viewing ability.

Only use hand movements (HM) or light perception (PL) when the vision is just that. A V/VA or HM or less has no functional vision and is not likely to improve with visual aids. Patients with this level of acuity may need further referral for sensory assistance.

A V/VA of 1/120, however, may benefit with the very high-powered LVAs for survival reading.

Record binocular acuity/preferred eye

Where there is a difference in acuity between the eyes, establish which is the eye the patient is most likely to use. It is not always the eye with the better acuity.

A previously amblyopic or squinting eye, which now retains the better acuity, will not necessarily be the preferred or fixating eye. The patient may still use the eye with the lower acuity, particularly if there has been a long-standing squint. This will have implications when prescribing magnification.

Patients with nystagmus (e.g. congenital idiopathic or nystagmus associated with a condition such as albinism) will often demonstrate a significant improvement in binocular acuity compared to monocular acuities. During refraction, allow the patient to adopt whatever posture they feel is most comfortable. Nystagmus patients may also exhibit a null point. This is the point at which the nystagmus is dampened, the visual acuity optimal, and thus the point at which the patient will have optimal discrimination during refraction. If the patient needs to

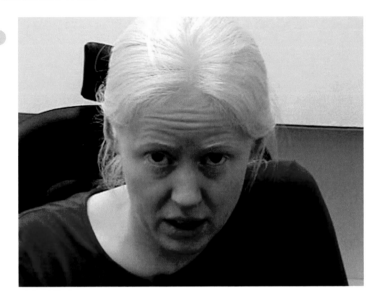

Figure 3.7 An abnormal head posture allows the patient to position their eyes at the null point

adopt an abnormal head posture to achieve the null point (Fig. 3.7), this may have implications on what type of low vision aid to use. It is also a good reason to avoid using a phoropter.

Eccentric viewing

Allow those patients who have adopted eccentric viewing due to a longstanding macular dystrophy/ARMD, etc., to use this during the refraction routine. In simulating the patient's visual behavior outside the consulting room, the practitioner may be more usefully able to influence the visual outcome.

Contrast sensitivity and glare

It is increasingly standard procedure to measure contrast sensitivity at this stage. Typically, this will be a Pelli–Robson score but may be an acuity reading taken with a low contrast chart as opposed to the high contrast score already measured. Many Bailey–Lovie charts have a reduced contrast version on their reverse side. Electronic charts, such as the City 2000, allow the contrast to be changed and acuity may be taken at several contrast levels. A reduced Pelli–Robson score or noticeable differences in acuity at different contrast levels should immediately highlight the need to incorporate specific advice about lighting in a management plan. Some centers have started using an external light source (such as a pentorch or a Brightness Acuity Test, or BAT) to see if there is an influence on acuity. Though not essential and difficult to quantify accurately, such an approach is simple and often very effective at simulating the detrimental effect glare may have on a patient's vision.

Cover test: distance and near

- Use large targets. Use whatever is appropriate to the level of vision and acuity. The measurement taken will be gross: knowledge of the fixing eye is important when considering the use of monocular units.
- Acquired defects can become divergent with time. This is often seen in those patients who have been referred for cataract surgery several years after the eye has become divergent. In such cases, intractable diplopia may occur.

Adaptations to the routine

Establishing distance refraction and acuity

Contrary to expectation, refracting patients with low vision is often more simple and quicker than for patients with normal acuity. The number of check tests which can be done are significantly fewer. Below are listed a few tips for a simple refraction.

Use larger steps

A patient with acuity of 2/60 will not be able to appreciate a difference of ±0.25. Therefore, use steps appropriate for the level of V/VA.

For example, ±1.00 spheres, ±1.00 DC cross-cyl.

Remember the limitations of subjective responses both due to the visual impairment and the patient's psychological adaptability.

Refract at a closer working distance

The chart of choice may be presented at 3 m or any other suitable distance: 1, 2 or 3 m. The benefits of this have already been discussed.

However, if the test chart and object of regard are closer than 6 m then the refraction obtained might not be accurate for viewing a target in the far distance. This will have a bearing on the final prescription.

For example, an eye that is looking at an object at 2 m will need an adjustment of 0.50D to the final prescription, i.e. if the patient was found to have a prescription of +1.75D at 2 m, then the final distance refraction will be adjusted to +1.25D. Arguably, this small difference will have little impact on a patient with poor visual acuity, and often it may be desirable to leave the patient overcorrected for distance. As acuity reduces it is often found that the patient looks into the distance rarely and objects at arms' length become more important. Similarly, it is not uncommon to leave the patient overcorrected for a close television viewing distance.

However, an adjustment of 1.00D while refracting an eye at 1 m may have more of an impact on the patient's distance acuity.

The one time it is important to have an accurate distance prescription is when the patient is using a fixed focus stand magnifier (see Chapter 5). If the lens to object distance of a fixed focus stand magnifier is set at the focal length of the magnifier's plus lens, f_1, then the emergent vergence entering the patient's eye will be parallel. This means that the patient will view the object as if it were a distant object, set at infinity. Therefore, any distance refractive error will need to be corrected.

If the patient had been refracted at 1 m and prescribed the correction found at this distance then they have theoretically been 'over-plussed' by +1.00D. If the patient were then to look through the stand magnifier then the image would remain out of focus, but may find that the image comes clearer if they were to pick the device up, turn it over and move the lens closer in towards the page, thereby turning the incident vergence from parallel to divergent, which the +1.00D will now correct.

Large refractive errors and cylindrical corrections

Correction of a significant refractive error or large cylindrical correction is still important despite no subjective improvement in central VA. A patient with a central scotoma may still prefer to wear the full correction to improve peripheral image quality.

Secondly, when prescribing near devices, in particular fixed vergence stand magnifiers or telescopic units, the full correction will become relevant. Magnification of an already poor quality image will be made even worse if a cylinder is not corrected.

Use a pinhole (PH) to check as usual. Corneal problems, which improve significantly with a PH, may justify a contact lens trial. A word of warning here. On occasions where the main cause of impairment is loss of media clarity (such as corneal, vitreous or lens disease) the visual improvement gained with the pinhole may not be repeatable with lenses and optical appliances, leaving the patient forever in search of the vision gained through the pinhole and unhappy with the aids prescribed.

Establishing near acuity

It is well understood that the measurement of reading performance in visually impaired patients should not be restricted to recording N-point notation.[25,34] When assessing the use of magnifiers, reading speeds and threshold should be taken into consideration.

Many practitioners find it useful to be able to estimate the expected near visual ability based on the distance acuity. This has several advantages. It allows the practitioner to direct the patient to a realistic starting target size (too small will frustrate, too large will slow down the assessment), it allows the practitioner to begin to think in terms of the expected level of magnification required for a task, and it also gives useful information about the patient's motivation. If a patient is expected to be able to read N12 (on the basis of a distance reading of 6/36), then if they fail to see any near target it might be remembered that this may be an indication that the patient has given up reading and is not willing to interpret the blurred near target presented to him. Near logMAR scores for a 25 cm card will reflect the same scores for the 4 meter distance chart. For Snellen acuity at 6 meters, a rough approximation using equivalent triangles allows one to predict a near N number of one-third the denominator (N12 at 25 cm for the 6/36 target). Though useful, this is very approximate; as will be repeated again, conditions often affect distance and near acuities differently. For example, posterior subcapsular cataract or macular degeneration will often affect near vision more than distance, nystagmus often being the opposite to this (see Chapter 4).

When prescribing magnification it is worth remembering that the N point sizes are a simple progression. N10 is twice the size of N5; N18 is three times larger than N6. A patient with a near acuity of N24 would, theoretically, need approximately 5× magnification to see N5. This, as will later be explained, may not be the best way to determine how much magnification a patient will need, but it will give an approximation only.

Record near working distances

It is essential to record all near working distances with visually impaired patients. A tape measure is essential kit! Quite often a patient will be adopting a working distance close to or within the focal length of the plus lens magnifier. The patient may find the working distance acceptable for low-powered plus lenses; however, the lens–object working distance of a high-powered plus lens will be significantly shorter. For example, maximum magnification of a 2.5× plus lens (10D) will be achieved with a small working distance of 10 cm.

Furthermore, if a patient explains that he has recently found his vision to be better without his bifocals, then record this on the record card. A −4D myope will have a working distance of approximately 25 cm, equivalent to his/her far point. Similarly, a −10D myope may have found an unaided vision of N5 when holding text at a 10 cm working distance. This is similar to the patient above, using a +10D spectacle magnifier. Encouraging the −10D myopic patient to adopt a close working distance may be all that is necessary for him rather than prescribing an expensive, complicated LVA. The effective 10D 'addition' will give them $2^{1}/_{2}×$ more magnification compared to the convention of a 25 cm working distance.

The low vision assessment in children

The aim of the low vision practice is to develop the child's visual abilities to his absolute limit, and allow him/her to use normal materials in a normal environment, so far as it is possible. A low vision examination with a child will clearly have similarities to examining children generally. Younger children tend to have low attention spans and become bored easily. With little children it is important to establish good communication early in the assessment. How do they use their vision? For example, children with very low vision may be learning Braille and touch-typing.

Questions will be directed to either the child or the parents and will depend on the child's age and whether there are other disabilities that may have a bearing on how the examination is conducted. Wherever possible, all should be included in the initial discussion, although the emphasis is for the child to be relaxed enough to lead and to allow for an honest and open account of his or her visual needs, where appropriate. Therefore, ask the child directly, and work quickly. However, have a relaxed attitude; it may take more than one visit.

Build up a picture of the child's home and educational needs, bearing in mind that there will be overlap between the two. The emphasis on any aid prescribed will be that it will have a wide range of uses; it is important not to label it as a reading instrument as is so easily done. Children typically will use the aid for almost anything, from shopping catalogs, maps, books, photos, jigsaws, etc. The list is endless. But told that it is an aid for reading, many children will use it for just that.

If a child is in special education or is receiving help from a peripatetic teacher of the visually impaired, he or she may already have been supplied with a magnifier. Establish what it is used for. If it is scratched then it probably has been well used. If it is still in its box, then probably the reverse is true. They may also have been given enlarged materials, use the blackboard very little and may even have a CCTV. A color CCTV is very useful for looking at picture books, even though color perception may often be seriously impaired.

Reading type

As previously mentioned, the McClure Children's Reading Chart ensures that the child's vision is measured rather than his or her reading ability. It is particularly useful to have one of these reading charts in a consulting room as it includes text for all age groups and for a larger range of acuities and also for a larger range of abilities.

Ask that the child bring to the examination any visual material that is causing difficulty, as perceived by both the child and the parents. It is often useful to see workbooks in current use and material that can be managed. All aids should be brought, whether used or not. These may include aids prescribed by other professionals.

It is worth noting that it is not only school tasks that cause problems. More time is spent at home, and it would be unwise to focus solely on difficulties encountered within the classroom. Build a picture of out of school activities, such as sports and games, toys and computer games, etc.

An accurate refraction is crucial. Modifications to the basic routine will be similar to those made for sighted children. Observe how the child reads, the position, working distance and posture. Some 5 year olds may be able to read. Some may not know their letters. It is unlikely that this is due to poor intellect and is more likely to be due to the age that the child started school.

Subjective results may or may not be useful. This is more dependent on age and cooperation. Retinoscopy should be accurate to within 0.50D. Any slight departure from the ideal refraction D is not going to make a crucial difference if the VA is low.

Do not assume a visually impaired child has a problem, as this is a current misconception. However, as school work progresses, regular visits will tackle potential problems head-on rather than allow them to interfere with development.

Prescribing for children

With children the consultation therefore tends to be more relaxed and less prescriptive. The device which works or which seems 'good enough' on the day is often the device that is taken home. There may be an emphasis on 'have a go at home and come back later and tell me how you got on'. Often there is one given for distance and one for near.

A child may not be able to assess many devices in the consulting room and subsequent visits will be needed to allow them to inspect additional or alternative equipment. Furthermore, although it is important to explain to parents and children the limitations of the device, it is also important to let the child explore with it and stress that it is an available option. By putting up boundaries such as 'use it for reading', then the child may use it for just that. If the child returns at the next visit, having been able to achieve at least one of his or her tasks, then the consultation is considered to be a success.

Follow up

Ideally, follow up should be rigorous, within 3–4 months of the initial consultation. A second relaxed consultation will include a chat about the device and what it has been used for. If it has come back scratched and worn then there are frequently some tales to tell. The range of tasks thought possible with any aid often increases sharply after a successful follow up with some children, from studying ants, biological dissection and 'Eye Spy Hide and Seek' to name but a few! Furthermore, if the child's acuity dramatically **improves** since the initial consultation, then it is safe to say that the aid has been used a lot and the child's skills have been developed.

As with all pediatric consultations, it is important to let them speak rather than the anxious parent. Nevertheless, it is important to include the parents in the discussion, perhaps after the initial information required has been gained. The parents' attitude to the device is very important, especially following an unsuccessful outcome. It may have been the limiting factor, and is one that may benefit from gentle encouragement.

Other parents are overprotective and restrict the child's development by doing too much for him or her. The optometrist must be able to recognize this and then refer on to the appropriate people, most especially if it seems that the parents have refused to accept that their child has a problem.

Examples of conditions requiring special consideration

Nystagmus

Congenital nystagmus is one of the most common causes of registration in children. It may occur without any other evidence of ocular pathology, or in association with another congenital ocular defect such as albinism or rod monochromatism. The amplitude of nystagmus and thus the patient's V/VA may drop with stress, fatigue, high illumination levels and dissociation. Alternatively, the amplitude may decrease with convergence when reading, or when the patient adopts a particular head posture.

If the amplitude of the nystagmus increases significantly, then it is likely that the visual acuity may drop and an accurate refractive end point will be more difficult to achieve. The practitioner must try to manage the nystagmus so that the patient may achieve maximum discrimination. Some tips for minimizing the effects are:

- Avoid occlusion by using fogging techniques to refract the patient binocularly. The patient is more likely to demonstrate better acuity with both eyes open than with one eye occluded.
- Allow the patient to adopt their normal head posture, even if this appears quite extreme (see Fig. 3.7). By allowing the patient to attain his/her null point, the nystagmus may be dampened to a degree where the pendular movements are checked and the VA achieved is at its maximum. A trial frame is better than a phoropter for ease of use.
- Patients often present with roughly equal VAs in each eye and due to the dampening of the nystagmus will often prefer binocular aids despite having poor or absent binocular function.
- Patients often demonstrate a better near visual acuity than what would have been expected from their distance visual acuity. Convergence for a near target may dampen the nystagmus significantly.

Albinism

There are two major types of albinism (total oculocutaneous and ocular), and the visual acuity varies between them.

A patient with albinism may present with astigmatic errors, squint, photophobia and nystagmus. Due to abnormal decussation of the chiasmal nerve fibers, albino patients do not demonstrate true binocular function.

All refractive errors should be fully corrected especially in children as often the full hypermetropic correction can significantly reduce or eliminate the need for near aids. Nearly all albino children can achieve N8 or better with simple refractive correction. By accommodating, the children merely hold the reading material close to gain the necessary 'magnification', the associated convergence may also dampen their nystagmus.

Albinos are photosensitive due to the reduction or complete lack of pigment within the eye. A tint will always be needed out of doors with additional UV protection. However, if glare sources are managed appropriately, then patients often prefer normal or near normal task illumination.

During refraction, those who are severely photosensitive may benefit from reducing the background room illumination slightly or turning off the illumination from within an internally illuminated test chart.

Congenital cataracts: aphakic children

Early diagnosis of congenital cataracts is vital (Fig. 3.8). All newborn children will have been checked for a clear red ophthalmoscopy reflex within the first few days of life by either a pediatrician or GP.

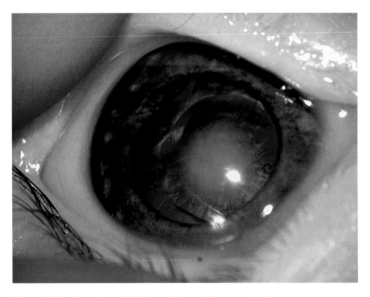

Figure 3.8 A nuclear (highly amblyogenic) congenital cataract (Reproduced with permission from Harvey & Gilmartin, *Paediatric Optometry*, Butterworth-Heinemann)

If there has been early surgical intervention there may be a chance of binocular function. Frequent refraction is then very important since the level of hypermetropia drops quite rapidly as the eye develops during the first few years of life. At present, few children are pseudophakic, although there are several who wear contact lenses from an early age.

With a clear reflex and no accommodative effort, objective refraction can be very accurate. A satisfactory end point is readily achieved with even the smallest of children by working directly on axis. However, a severe uniocular cataract imposes difficult management, with contact lenses providing the best correction and spectacles an alternative.

For the majority of aphakic children a bifocal with a +4.00D−+6.00D addition is adequate, as they will naturally have working distances shorter than those of adults. Moreover, the 30% larger image size has its advantages.

Age-related macular degeneration

ARMD is by far the largest single cause of visual impairment that is encountered in general ophthalmic practice. Approximately 70% of people included on the Blind and Partial Sight Registers for the United Kingdom are over 75 years of age.[1] Macular degeneration is the most common cause, accounting for approximately half of registered cases.[1]

Patients present with varying degrees of central scotomas, with associated acuities from 6/6 − PL. Peripheral fields remain intact, and patients often find this fact confusing when discussing their symptoms. It is a common grievance that they are unable to see the headlines of a newspaper and yet can see a small spider walk across the carpet, or an aeroplane high in the sky.

Patients with a recent central (positive) scotoma may noticeably move their head a lot during testing, often complaining that the lenses are 'smudgy'. It is less likely that they will adopt an eccentric viewing position so early on in the disease process. Indeed, they may never achieve this at all without training. Consequently, refraction results may present a discrepancy between the near and distance VAs. A patient with relatively good distance acuity may have an anomalous poor near acuity.

However, patients with long-standing scars may have adopted an eccentric viewing technique naturally and often return to the low vision clinic with an apparent improvement on their near acuity.

4
Determining and prescribing magnification

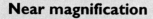
Near magnification

Using the charts

As previously mentioned, there is also a direct mathematical relationship between letter size notations on the Times New Roman Faculty of Ophthalmologists reading chart:

> N12 is half the size of N24
> N6 is half the size of N12
> N9 is twice the size of N4.5

By using this method: if a patient sees N10 with their current spectacles then one can assume that 2× magnification is required to see N5.

This method is quick and useful for patients with relatively good distance and near acuities. However, this is not an accurate method to use when the VA is poor as there will be several other factors affecting the result.

The 'divide by three' rule

This 'rule' gives an estimation of near acuity based on the distance Snellen acuity. For example, if the distance acuity is 6/24, then the expected near acuity should be 24/3 = N8 at a working distance of 25 cm (assuming any relevant near correction is in place). Near logMAR scores for a 25 cm card will reflect the same scores for the 4 meter distance chart, so such an estimate is not necessary.

It must be stressed, however, that this is just estimation as, in practice, patients with low vision rarely bear out this relationship exactly. Reading acuity does not correlate well with distance Snellen visual acuity and significantly less so with visually impaired patients. Patients with ARMD, for example, will often demonstrate a significantly reduced near acuity than what would be expected from their distance acuity, due to the presence of a central scotoma. Posterior subcapsular cataracts can also give anomalous results. The cataract is close to the nodal point of the eye and despite relatively good distance acuity, the near VA can be quite poor. Furthermore, pupillary constriction will enhance the influence of scotomata and opacities. In other cases it may offer a better depth of focus, allowing better near acuity than might be expected.

Reading is also a complex visual task; if words are used as a target then it is easy for a patient to guess subsequent words on a page from the meaning of the text.

The low vision routine

The technique below is a well-established methodical routine, which is an extremely useful method for assessing required magnification. It gives a good foundation upon which the rest of the consultation is based. Most low vision practitioners will use this method in some format or another.

1. Begin by establishing the patient's baseline near acuity with a +4.00D addition at 25 cm (25 cm being the focal length of the +4.00D lens).
2. If the level of VA is much less than that which the patient needs to undertake the desired task, then start by increasing the addition in the trial frame until the desired acuity is met, usually in +4.00D steps. For closer acuity to the target acuity, use smaller steps (1 or 0.5D steps). For each addition, note the acuity, the working distance and some note of the ease of task or quality of the viewing for the patient.
3. When the desired near visual acuity is met, the magnification of the high reading addition thus demonstrated will give the practitioner a starting point magnification with which to demonstrate the device of choice, such as a hand magnifier.
4. Explain the reduced working distance, and demonstrate the effect of illumination (Fig. 4.1).
5. If the patient finds the closer working distance unacceptable, then they may need encouragement to try a spectacle magnifier. Instead, try demonstrating alternative aids around the calculated magnification.
6. Record patient handling, motivation and achieved VA with each aid shown (for example, 'N12 at 12 cm with +8.00 add, difficulty with working distance').
7. With higher magnification, it is important to demonstrate that an increase in magnification means a smaller field of view, not to mention a smaller magnifier.
8. A telescopic service may be demonstrated if required (Fig. 4.2).

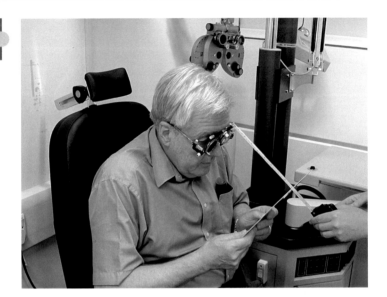

Figure 4.1 Assessing performance with increasing reading addition

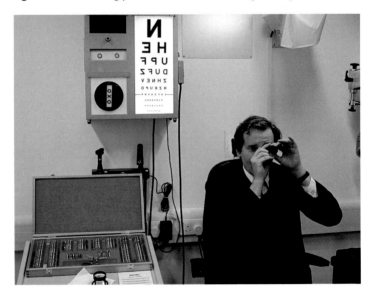

Figure 4.2 Assessing handling and use of a monocular telescope

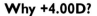
Why +4.00D?

Magnification, in the above example, is merely the comparison of the old object distance to the new object distance. For example, if we cannot see the number plate of a car, we move up closer to it, the retinal image size increasing all the time. If a patient moves in towards a television by half the total distance, then the image of the television, or the retinal image size, will double the size. This is termed **relative distance magnification**.

$$\text{Magnification} = \frac{\text{Old object distance}}{\text{New object distance}}$$

When establishing near magnification, as in the above method, by convention, we call the old object distance 25 cm. This is often termed 'the least distance of distinct vision', as convergence is possible at this distance so it represents a sensible baseline distance on which to assess near visual function (in a world of long-armed people, 50 cm might have been adopted giving us a magnification formula of $M = F/2$).

For example, if a patient needed to bring the print in to 12.5 cm in order for it to be seen, then the retinal image size is 2× larger than it was when it had been held at 25 cm, our conventional starting point:

$$M = \frac{25}{12.5} = \times 2$$

What the lenses do is to merely focus the retinal image of the object at the given distance, in this case a +4.00D addition for a 25 cm working distance, and a +8.00D addition for a 12.5 cm working distance. Alternatively, the patient may wish to use their accommodative effort, if they have it. Thus, it is typical for a visually impaired child to hold text very close in order to achieve 'magnification' of the print or object.

From the above equation, and on the assumption that 25 cm is the conventional 'old' object distance, we derive the magnification formula,

$$M = F/4$$

+4.00D at 25 cm	1×	(by convention)
+8.00D at 12 cm	2×	
+10.00D at 10 cm	2.5×	
+20.00D at 5 cm	5×	

From this, we call +4.00D add **unit magnification**. Each successive addition of another 4 diopters adds another unit of magnification.

From the practical viewpoint, this method quickly establishes the estimated magnification a patient will require to see an object of a given size, most typically, the printed text.

Too many practitioners get obsessive about +4.00D being the starting point when ascribing the magnification a patient may achieve with any particular aid. It is important to remember that from the patient point of view, the magnification they will achieve with any particular aid will be based on how much larger the target may look with the aid they leave the practice with compared to its apparent size when they first entered the practice. For example, many patients will attend wearing a +2.50D addition in their existing bifocals. If they are subsequently offered a +10.00D addition for reading, convention based on the +4.00D magnification derivation would dictate that this represented a magnification of 2.5 times. However, relative to the initial add the patient was wearing, this represents a magnification of four times (10/2.5 or a reduction in the working distance from 40 cm with their old add to 10 cm with their new add). This is perhaps more useful in that it represents the change perceived by the patient rather than that derived from a physical concept.

Mr T

Refraction

$+3.00/-1.00 \times 165 = 6/24^{+2}$ $\qquad$ $+4.00/-1.25 \times 180 = 6/60$

$\qquad$ logMAR 0.54 $\qquad\qquad$ logMAR 1.00

$\qquad$ Add +2.75 = N10 at 30 cm $\qquad$ Add +2.75 = N24 at 32 cm

$\qquad$ Add +4.00 = N6 at 25 cm $\qquad$ Add +4.00 = N24 at 25 cm

$\qquad$ Add +6.00 = N5 fair at 17 cm

$\qquad$ Add +8.00 = N5 well at 12 cm

- Although he appreciated the significant improvement to his near acuity, Mr T complained that the short working distance was unacceptable to him. This is not at all unusual. It is typically the younger patients, who have been accommodating to hold work close, who are more tolerant of the shorter working distances.
- The power required to improve his vision to N5 (approximately a +6.00D or +8.00D lens) is the power of his own magnifier. As would be expected, it is the poor quality image, caused by the scratches on the lens, which is resulting in an underachievement in his near VA.
- By using the formula $M + F/4$ by convention, one would expect Mr T to require a 1.5×–2× magnifier to improve his near acuity to N5.

Mrs M

Refraction (RE)

$-3.50/-3.00 \times 155 = 6/60^{+1}$

$\qquad$ logMAR 0.98

Add +4.00 $\quad$ = $\quad$ N24 at 25 cm

Add +8.00 $\quad$ = $\quad$ N14 at 13 cm

Add +12.00 $\quad$ = $\quad$ N12 at 8 cm

Add +16.00 $\quad$ = $\quad$ N12 at 6 cm

Add +20.00 $\quad$ = $\quad$ N10 at 5 cm

Add +25.00 $\quad$ = $\quad$ N10 at 4 cm poor, unable to maintain focus at close working distance.

- The nucleosclerotic cataract in the RE had caused a myopic shift of approximately −1.00D. This would have accounted for her 40 cm working distance with her current bifocals. The working distance should correspond to the focal length of the plus lens in the trial frame. If it does not, and there is a significant discrepancy, then it is possible that the original distance prescription was inaccurate. Exceptions to this rule are when there is a tiny pupil, as a consequence, perhaps, of pupil miosed under the influence of pilocarpine medication, resulting in an improvement in the depth of focus. A second factor may be a difference in refractive index of the media.
- Mrs M did not appreciate the improvement in her distance vision.
- Mrs M finds the central scotoma due to the macular hole difficult to overcome. As a consequence of this, she appears to have a disproportionate improvement in her near acuity with increased magnification. She may benefit from eccentric viewing training.
- Currently, she would require a minimum of 5× magnification to improve her near acuity to N10.

One advantage of using this step-by-step method is that for each additional unit of magnification added in the trial frame, the patient should see an improvement, which does help in restoring confidence. However, there are many patients who resist the close working distance that each additional lens brings, and this could indicate a challenge if a spectacle magnifier is to be prescribed.

It is also worth mentioning here that patients with a recent central scotoma often do not show an improvement with each addition. This may indicate the need for eccentric viewing training. Mrs M appears to be demonstrating that need, for example.

The above method describes the minimum magnification required to view a high contrast near acuity test card, of predetermined size. However, the actual amount of magnification that is actually prescribed will depend on several other factors:

1. Reading speed required for the task: i.e. whether the task involves a degree of fluency or sustained reading, or whether the task is merely a spot check.

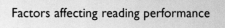

2. The contrast of the task.
3. The patient's visual field.

Factors affecting reading performance

Reading rates and acuity reserve[25,34–42,47]

During the previous 'work-up', the minimum magnification required for a patient to reach the target acuity has been estimated.

While this minimum amount of magnification may be all that is necessary to look at a washing machine dial or a can label, it is not possible to work at or on this threshold for sustained or fluent reading tasks, such as reading the newspaper or a novel.

For sustained reading, more magnification will be required than what has previously been estimated. In other words, the patients will keep a degree of acuity *in reserve*.

This **acuity reserve** is calculated as the ratio of the target acuity to the patient's threshold acuity (with a device). For sustained reading tasks, this ratio has been estimated to be between 2:1 and 3:1.[25,34]

For example, if a patient needs to be able to read newsprint successfully (N8 approximately), then we need to consider sufficient magnification for him or her to be able to read at least N4 or better. If the patient is given an aid with which he can only achieve N8, then it is less likely that reading newsprint will be sustained for any length of time and the outcome will be deemed less successful. For logMAR scoring, where there is a multiplication factor of around 1.26 times between lines, a useful guide to prescribing an adequate acuity reserve is to allow a threshold acuity of 0.2 less than the required target size (for example, to read fluently 0.4 size print, offer sufficient magnification to just see 0.2 size print).

However, for survival or spot reading, an acuity reserve of 1:1 is all that is considered necessary, and a patient can have a magnifier that allows him or her to work close to threshold. Usually in such cases, giving an unnecessarily strong magnifier

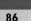
would compromise the patient's field of view and further reduce the working distance of the task.

Reading rates

Whittaker and Lovie-Kitchen[34] demonstrated that as the print size reduces towards threshold acuity, the reading speed slows down.

Similarly, a patient's reading rate will continue to improve suprathreshold until a threshold performance is reached. For spot checks an estimated reading rate of 40 words per minute (wpm) is needed. For sustained reading, this reading rate will increase to approximately 150 wpm. An impaired reading speed, for whatever reason, may impair the patient's comprehension of the text.

MNREAD Acuity Charts

In 1989 Legge *et al.*[37] introduced the Minnesota Low-vision Reading Test, a computer-generated system for measuring reading speeds. Later, a simplified version was created for use in clinical practice called the MNREAD Acuity Charts.[41,42]

The MNREAD Acuity Charts are continuous text reading acuity charts for normal and low vision (see Chapter 3). They can be used to assess how reading performance depends on print size. Three measures of reading performance are obtained:

1. *Reading acuity*—the smallest print that can just be read.
2. *Maximum reading speed*—the reading speed when performance is not limited by print size.
3. *Critical print size*—the smallest print that supports the maximum reading speed.

Contrast sensitivity and contrast reserve

It is well understood that a single visual acuity measurement does not give a complete description of the patient's ability to detect large objects and low contrasts in the real world.[48,49] In fact, what it does measure is the ability to see the highest spatial frequency at maximum contrast. This is only one small part of a person's actual visual environment. Contrast sensitivity measurements are considered to be a more accurate measure of a patient's visual function.[35,36,48–54]

For example, a reduced sensitivity to contrast in a patient with an otherwise good Snellen acuity may explain his or her difficulty with steps and kerbs. The object may be large enough to detect, but the subtle difference in contrast between one step and the next may be below the patient's contrast threshold and therefore he or she will be unable to see it.

The contrast sensitivity function (CSF) is the reciprocal of the contrast detection threshold for sine wave gratings of variable spatial frequency (cycles/degree) and contrast.[48,49] Measurement of the CSF is classically measured with an oscilloscope system generating sine wave gratings. Patients who have been found to have a low-contrast threshold for detection of a sine wave grating indicates very high contrast sensitivity. This means that they have been able to detect the grating when it has been presented with low or minimal contrast.

A patient's ability to detect contrast is assessed frequently in those with a visual impairment. It is used to identify patients who report a relatively normal visual acuity yet reveal subjective visual difficulties, for example, in detecting large objects. Secondly, the assessment of contrast sensitivity has also been shown to be of significant value in assessment of the patient's reading performance and predicting the success of using low vision aids.[25,34]

The resolution of a sine wave grating is a simple, low-level task. It does not involve the more complex task of recognizing and naming letters. Despite this, measurements of a patient's CSF using the traditional oscilloscope are expensive and difficult to reproduce in a clinical practice setting. Consequently, a number of clinical tests have been produced for use in clinical practice. These include:

1. Sinusoidal gratings at a limited number of spatial frequencies (e.g. Vistech VCTS chart).
2. Low contrast letter acuity charts (Bailey–Lovie, Pelli–Robson charts, or reproduced using the City 2000 and City 2000 PRO).

Bailey–Lovie chart

On the reverse of a standard high-contrast Bailey–Lovie chart, there is a low-contrast letter logMAR chart. The patient is asked to read letters of decreasing size at both levels of contrasts. The smallest letter size that can be read at a given contrast level is representative of the cut-off spatial frequency at that level, and by measuring this at the two contrast levels of 100 and 10%, respectively, the difference is an indication of the right-hand slope of the CSF.[51]

A normally sighted viewer will not show a significant reduction in acuity at the lower contrast level. However, a disproportional poor acuity for the low-contrast letters may be found in patients with glaucoma or multiple sclerosis.

Pelli–Robson low contrast letter chart and contrast threshold[35,55,56]

The print quality that we read every day tends to vary significantly in contrast. For example, a computer can generate a 100% contrast, a laser printer 90%, a paperback novel 75% and a newspaper between 60 and 70%.

The Pelli–Robson chart (Fig. 4.3) is considered to be a simple and efficient way to establish a patient's contrast threshold within a clinical setting. It is quick, simple to use and is easily understood by the patient. By altering the logCS scoring to Michelson

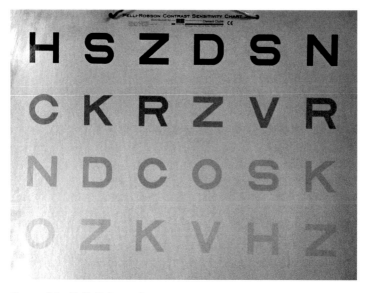

Figure 4.3 Pelli–Robson chart

contrast values, it can be appreciated that an eye with
a threshold of 10% performs twice as well as an eye with
a 20% threshold.[25]

Whittaker and Lovie-Kitchen[34] have defined **contrast
reserve as** the ratio between the print contrast and the patient's
measured contrast threshold. A contrast reserve required for
sustained reading tasks and spot checks has been
estimated to be:

- Fluent reading 10:1.
- Spot reading 3:1.

For example, if a patient has a contrast threshold of 11%, and the
contrast of the print that the patient needs to read is 75%, the
contrast reserve will be ($^{75}/_{11} \sim$ 6.8). As this is well below
that estimated for sustained reading, the patients may find

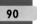

limited success. This patient, however, may benefit from an aid for spot checks unless the text is enhanced by other methods.

Visual field defects[57–60]

Despite a good acuity reserve and contrast threshold, the patients may still never achieve high fluent reading due to the size and location of a visual field defect.

An Amsler chart (Fig. 4.4) will assist in obtaining an assessment of the central 10 degrees and any irregularities found can be located, mapped and latterly accounted for when prescribing magnification or dispensing a visual aid.

Field size

Studies have indicated that for spot checks, a minimum of two characters must be visible, whereas a minimum of four to six characters must be visible before the patient may be able to obtain sustained fluency. However, there has been a wide variation in the methods used to determine this value.

Steady eye strategy (SES) involves keeping the eye still and moving the text from right to left. **Eccentric viewing** (EV) is a technique by which the patient will view an object eccentric to the fovea, termed the **preferred retinal location** (PRL). Both techniques are used in patients with central scotomata and can be used either together or independently.

Eccentric viewing is usually established at an early age in patients with a congenital macular loss. So much so, that often the patient may not be aware that they are looking to the side of the object, or not aware that they are not looking directly at an individual while talking to them.[61] However, in elderly patients, eccentric viewing techniques are rarely obtained spontaneously and only under specific conditions such as a well-defined, positive scotoma. However, the quality of most central lesions will vary

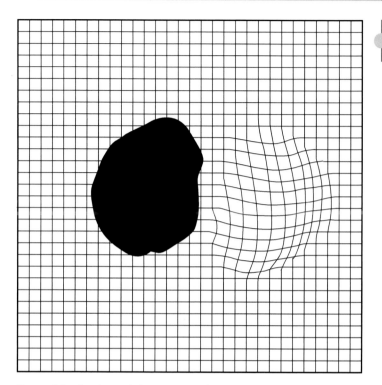

Figure 4.4 Amsler grid showing central scotoma and distortion. Note the displacement of the scotoma to the left, which may have less effect on reading than a similar defect to the right

from one point to the next and are rarely well defined and, therefore, in most cases, training may be necessary.

As the text is moved in SES, the eye can be trained so that the letters will fall on a predetermined PRL, which may have already been predetermined with an Amsler chart (Fig. 4.4). Resolution of the PRL will drop sharply, the more eccentric to the fovea. Magnification may improve the ability to see the letters, but the patient may still not be able to read successfully since there are now fewer letters on the PRL at any one time.

Hemianopic defects also have an impact on reading performance, and often represent a considerable challenge to both practitioner and patient. Defects on the right side of the visual field will have an impact on reading from left to right. Defects on the left side of the visual field can cause problems in locating the start of the next line.

Various therapies can be tried, including the use of prisms and mirrors, and altering the orientation of the text, each with a degree of success in a well motivated patient.[62] One well known approach, which is occasionally successful with a right hemi-field loss, is for a person who normally reads from left to right to adapt to reading upside down.

Lighting and reading performance

More light is needed with older subjects.[63] Age related miosis and media changes in a 60-year-old subject are some of the reasons why there is three times less light reaching the retina compared to that of a 20-year-old subject. Therefore it follows that more light will be needed for elderly patients compared to younger patients. If pathology causes light scatter, as with media-related disease, the impact of varying light will be significant. Furthermore, the reduction in ability to distinguish different contrast targets with, for example, macular degeneration means that contrast enhancement by increasing lighting further is often necessary.

Visual task performance improves with light. However, an excess of light will cause discomfort glare, at which point the performance may plateau, and then there will be an initial decrease in performance until the point of cut-off as the glare becomes disabling.

Patients with macular degeneration benefit from having a significant increase in the amount of light available to them. Several studies have put this value as an additional increase of 1000 lux, although some studies have suggested values as high as an additional increase of 15,000 lux. Lighting should be localized and close to the page, but removable. The results of several studies [64–66] have resulted in the Chartered Institute of Building Services Engineers in the UK (CIBSE UK) recommendations that visually impaired patients require approximately 10 times more illuminance compared to age-matched normals.[65] Patients in some cases are able to read with lower magnification.[67,68] It is suggested that the receptive field size may decrease at higher levels of illumination, i.e. the size of the central scotoma will be smaller in relation to the size of the print.[25]

Prescribing strategies

After determining the magnification required for the task, and making an assessment of visual performance, it is important to have a clear strategy for prescribing. Rumney[25] differentiates patients into three distinct groups on the basis of their threshold visual performance:

1. Limited or no survival reading potential.
2. Survival reading potential but limited likelihood of fluency.
3. Clear survival reading potential with fluent reading possible if motivated.

It is important to start with the survival reading first to assist independence. Following any success here, then fluent reading may be introduced later. More than one appointment may be necessary, with motivation being a strong indicator for success in those patients who have indicated a potentially good reading performance. Often a patient will return having tried the aid at home for a while and, pleased with its initial success with survival or spot reading, is motivated to take things onto another level.

The list below gives several factors that are relevant when considering the design of a device to demonstrate to the patient.

- Does the patient need a device that is hands free or spectacle mounted?
- Does the patient have the ability to hold hand steady?
- Does the patient have ease of handling or is there any factor such as arthritis that will affect the ability to hold a hand-held device?

- Is there a need for a flat surface?
- Is a close working distance acceptable?
- Is there a need for portability?
- Is additional lighting necessary?
- Is the cosmesis important to the patient?
- Will there be training involved?
- Is cost important?

Mr T

Aids demonstrated:

With bifocals

+8D aspheric hand mag. = N6 well, good handling ('too dark')
+8D aspheric hand mag. = N5 part ('too small')
+11.5D hand mag. = N4 well ('too small')
+12D aspheric hand mag. = N4 well (prefers this, but a bit shaky)
+12D aspheric stand mag. = N4 with ease ('too big and clumsy')

Without bifocals

+11.5D hand mag. = N4 well (improved field by holding closer to eye)
Prescribed +11.5D hand mag. for N10 books (acuity reserve
N10:N4 = 2.5:1) and cooking instructions
Advice given on lighting

Review 3/12

Mrs M

Aids demonstrated:

With new prescription,

+20D Hand magnifier = N14 fair. Handling fair
+28D Hand magnifier = dislikes this, would not try
+20D Stand magnifier = N10 fair, but 'too dark'
+20D Illuminated stand magnifier = N8 fair
+24D Illuminated stand magnifier = N8 well. Good handling
+28D Illuminated stand magnifier = N6 well

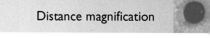

Prefers to try 24D illuminated stand magnifier for now. Prescribed for short near tasks: recipes, personal mail (acuity reserve 1:1)

Will review at 3/12. Referred for social services information, etc.

Distance magnification

Prescribing magnification for distance is less frequent and tends to be for younger, more mobile patients. Examples of commonly aired problems include:

- Train indicator boards.
- Street names.
- Supermarket aisles.
- Bus numbers.
- Scoreboards at football or cricket grounds.
- Galleries and museums.
- Recognizing people across the road.

However, less mobile patients may still request distance consideration. It is not uncommon to have requests for help with:

- Watching the grandchildren at the end of the garden.
- Television.
- Theatre.

Calculation is straightforward and prescribing more so due to the limitation in both the range of magnification and the design of devices available. All distance devices are telescopic in nature as they exploit angular magnification as opposed to relative distance magnification.

Once the patient's distance refraction has been determined, then the amount of magnification required to see an object is a simple comparison between the patient's current acuity and the size of the object that he or she wishes to view. Hence, if a patient's acuity is 6/60, then theoretically they should require 10× magnification to achieve 6/6. In reality, however, most patients will not have the need to obtain a 6/6 acuity. It is more common to settle for acuity of approximately 6/12, as this will usually suffice for most of the examples stated above. Many patients usually cope better with the less strong magnification, as they prefer the slightly wider field of view and more stable image position with a weaker telescope.

However, a current complaint has been directed at the recently upgraded indicator boards at railway and bus stations; despite the excellent computer-generated graphics and superb contrast, it is not possible to see the text unless the individual is standing square on to the screen. In addition, the text is so small that it may be necessary for the patient to achieve an acuity greater than 6/9 through a distance device and especially at peak travel times when access closer to the screen may not be possible.

There are essentially two fundamental ways in which a patient can achieve distance magnification:

1. Move closer to the object
By decreasing the viewing distance and moving closer to the object, the retinal image size will increase (relative distance magnification). Of course, in reality, this may not always be possible.

However, most patients, who have tried using a telescopic device for watching television, often revert back to sitting closer, as the latter, in most cases, is preferable.

Magnification of the screen is obtained by decreasing the viewing distance. Sitting half the distance closer than normal will increase the new retinal image size by two-fold. A small addition for the shorter viewing distance (for example, +0.50D for a 2 m distance, +1.00D addition for a 1 m viewing distance, etc.) may be perceivable to the patient, depending on his or her acuity.

Often, following lengthy discussion, it is not uncommon to find that the patient has been previously avoiding sitting so close to the television for fear of causing harm to his or her eyesight. The low vision practitioner has the time and authority to dispel such myths.

2. Use a telescope (Fig. 4.2)
The use of a distance telescope avoids the need for altering the working distance. Most commonly these devices are prescribed

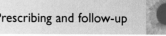

for use out of doors as an aid to mobility, for example, train indicator boards and street signs. The object will be stationary; there has been limited success in the use of a telescopic aid for a moving object, such as a bus, due to the severely restricted field of view: most distance telescopes have a field of view of approximately 7 degrees. Moving targets are easier to see through a telescope when approaching or receding rather than tracked from the side.

Mr T

Distance telescopes (right eye)
Shown 1.8× finger ring telescope = 6/12 easily
Shown Eschenbach 4× monocular telescope = 6/9 difficulty locating object

Prescribed finger ring telescope for local cricket matches

Prescribing and follow-up

At the initial consultation, it is important to have a strategy for prescribing, as outlined above. It is usually not possible to deal with all requests during the first visit, and similarly, it is not possible to eliminate all fears. It is unlikely that a patient who initially appears satisfied and reassured after the first visit has not revealed the whole picture.

It is important to remember that in the same way it is not always necessary to achieve 6/6, it is not always necessary to achieve N5. There is little point in giving the patient an excess of magnification to achieve N5 when N12 will do. In Mr T's case, he needed something to read novels with, so acuity of N4 or N5 was necessary with the aid, in order to have an acuity reserve sufficient for sustained reading. However, if he had requested that he only wished to read large print books (e.g. N18), then significantly less magnification would have been all that was necessary. There then would have been an improvement in the field of view.

Generally the aid given will be the one that the patient performed best with on the day.

Leave the patient to try the aid at home for a while, and then bring them back to find out how they are managing, if the aid was indeed useful and if any new problems are arising.

5
Optical principles of low vision aids

contents continue

5

Optical principles of low vision aids

Prescribing the hardware

Once the level of magnification required for the task has been established, we then need to demonstrate aids of appropriate choice to meet the patient's needs. We will have already determined what it is that the patient wants to see (within reason), their expectations, and their motivation. We should also have determined the categories of aids that would be considered most appropriate for the task. For example, if the patient needs something to help him/her see the prices of goods in a supermarket, then a spectacle-mounted telescope is not a good choice.

Making the right choice

When prescribing an aid, we need to consider many different aspects of the patient's lifestyle. Table 5.1 is worth bearing in mind when choosing a device.

It is important to be able to narrow the initial choice of aid to a few, and to avoid the despair of going through a number of unsuitable devices, which may be upsetting for the patient.

Motivation: using a low vision aid

A picture of the patient's motivation will gradually emerge during the consultation. An elderly patient whose vision has dropped recently due to ARMD, or perhaps a patient who has 'given up on reading' for example, may initially require encouragement. They may be reluctant to try an aid even if it noticeably improves their visual acuity. Similarly, if we approach the consultation with any negativity then this will rub off on the patient. Always take a positive and encouraging view.

The final response to an aid will vary with the patient. Often patients with acquired disabilities may see the aid as a constant reminder that their vision is not as good as what it used to be. The patient with a congenital loss, however, may be quite different. To them, an aid may be considered an enhancement on their already normal situation.

Table 5.1 **Consider many different aspects of the patient's lifestyle when choosing a device**

The size and working distance of the task	Established during your routine, e.g. studying maps at a schoolroom desk, watching television at a distance of 1 m, reading large print books at a desk in local library
Hands-free/spectacle mounted	Does patient need to have hands free to hold a book/paper? Can they have the text mounted on a stand?
Ability to hold hand steady	Relates to hand-held devices: e.g. hand magnifiers and distance telescopes
Ease of handling	Are there any other factors that will contribute to the patient being unable to manage the device?
Need for a flat surface	E.g. large newspapers may need a larger surface. Reading packets and cans: avoid the use of a fixed focus stand magnifier
Acceptable cosmesis	Consider where the patient is going to use the device. In public?
Training involved	Can they cope with a high reading addition? Is eccentric viewing necessary? Will patient need to be shown how to use a hand-held telescope?
Environment	Using a LVA in public emphasizes a disability, e.g. a child at school may feel conspicuous using an aid in public
Close working distance acceptable	More acceptable with younger or highly motivated patients.

Continued

Table 5.1 **Consider many different aspects of the patient's lifestyle when choosing a device—cont'd**

Portability	Does the aid need to be portable?
Integral lighting	Halogen devices may need a mains supply
Cost	Will the aid be on loan or is it a private purchase? The cost may be a concern. NHS Voucher will not be applicable.

Classification of optical low vision aids

Spectacle magnifiers.
Hand magnifiers.
Stand magnifiers.
Telescopes (distance and near).
Electronic devices, CCTV, etc.

As a general rule, when prescribing low vision aids it is sensible to start at the beginning. By far the majority of low vision aids prescribed are simple hand and stand magnifiers. Spectacle high reading additions and telescopic devices are often more suited to more motivated patients.

Following the discussion on acuity reserve in Chapter 4 it follows that prescribing too much magnification will be unconstructive. The aim is to prescribe the **minimum** acceptable magnification with the **maximum** acceptable field of view wherever possible. Both field of view and working distance are rapidly compromised at increased levels of magnification.

It also follows that if a patient needs a hand magnifier to read large print books, they will require more magnification if they wanted to read newsprint. If the patient regularly carries out both tasks, then perhaps two different magnifiers would be sensible.

Spectacle magnifiers

The term 'spectacle magnifier' relates to a high plus lens or lenses worn in the spectacle plane. Generally, it is one thickness of refracting material before the eye (though it may be a compound lens if two or more lenses are cemented together) as opposed to two or more lenses separated by a space (which would be described as a telescope even if held in a spectacle frame). There are many ways that spectacle magnification may be achieved, and all are variations on a theme of 'stronger glasses'. These include, although not an exhaustive list:

'Ready-mades'

- For example, COIL aspheric–prismatic half-eyes. Up to +12.00D with 14∆ in (Fig. 5.1).
- Many hospital departments will also keep ready-readers up to +20.00D and one eye may be occluded to avoid binocular confusion.

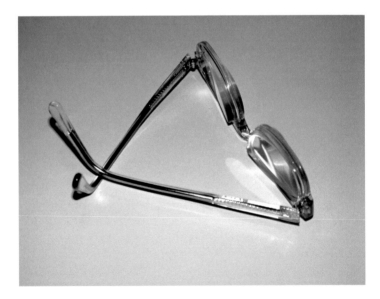

Figure 5.1 Spectacle magnifiers—note the base in prism

High-plus power single vision[69]

- Single vision lenticulars up to +45.00D.
- Single vision aspheric up to +20.00D.
- Aspheric hyperocular up to ×12 (+71.36D). These biconvex aspheric lenses allow high magnification while still maintaining a reasonable field of view and minimal distortion.

Sola bifocals

- Round segment bifocal additions from +4.00D to +16.00D.

Keeler trephined bifocal

- Small bifocal button screwed into plano-carrier lens.

Keeler advanced bifocal

- Button screwed into a carrier cemented onto the front surface of the lens so maintaining any cylindrical correction.
- Both these are found usually from 2× to 9× but may be obtained up to 15×.

Compound lenses or lens systems

Compound lenses are made up of more than one lens, usually cemented together in a carrier. They are often mistaken for telescopes; however, this is not the case as typically both lenses will have the same diameter and there will be no visible space between them. In the case of telescopes, the eyepiece lens and the objective lenses are of two different diameters, the former usually being the smaller of the two. The purpose of the compound lens system is to achieve higher levels of magnification without the significant aberrational effect that would occur in a high-powered single vision lens. Often the eyepiece and objective lenses of telescope are made up of compound lens systems. Magnification is available up to 20×, such as the Keeler 20× with light unit.

The need for occlusion

Patients with an asymmetrical loss of vision may find that the fellow eye (usually the one with the worse V/VA) 'interferes', and will prefer to close one eye. This seems particularly evident in patients with ARMD where the positive central scotoma of the fellow eye causes a disturbance. Here, a frosted lens or an occluder may be useful. A temporary measure can be obtained with the use of Blenderme, a semitransparent bandage tape readily available from pharmacists. It is often applied to fellow lens for a trial period before the frosted or Chavasse lens is ordered.

Binocularity and prismΔ incorporation

If a high-powered addition is given binocularly, increased convergence will be needed to avoid diplopia. For every diopter of focusing for near vision, whether by accommodation or lens addition, there is an associated one-meter angle of convergence. So, for any low vision patient viewing an object at 10 cm (e.g. +10.00D lens giving 2.5× magnification) 10 meter angles of convergence will have to be used to maintain binocular single vision. This value may be converted into prism diopters by multiplying the interpupillary distance in centimeters by the meter angle value.

> *Worked example*
> 1. For a patient with an interpupillary distance (PD) of 65 mm viewing at 1 m, the convergence required is 6.5Δ.
> 2. For a patient with PD of 65 mm viewing at 10 cm, the convergence required is 65Δ.

To allow for the extra convergence, adequate decentration or base-in prism should be worked, a rule-of-thumb being '1 mm in decentration of bifocal segment for each diopter of reading addition for each eye or, for single vision lenses, one prism diopter base-in ground on lenses for each diopter of reading addition in each eye'.

> *Worked example*
> For the patient with +10.00D addition and PD of 65 mm, 10 mm decentration should be given to each lens (or 10Δ base-in each eye if single vision).

Maintenance of binocularity above +12.00D is often difficult but not a significant problem, as usually a patient will have one very dominant eye. If high magnification and binocularity is essential, then a useful aid is a binocular near vision telescope. The units can be aligned such that their axes converge. An example of these is the Keeler 21, or long-tube telescope, which can be successfully mounted binocularly to achieve up to ×5 magnification at near.

Advantages and disadvantages of spectacle magnifiers

Many elderly patients, who have spent a lifetime with a book on their lap, often find the closer working distance of higher-powered spectacle magnifiers unacceptable. This may be as much a physical constraint in holding things so close with less depth of focus, as a psychological constraint that needs to be adapted to. It is also important to remember that reduced working distances also reduce illuminance. On the other hand, those patients who have lived with a congenital visual impairment have a higher success rate, having previously used accommodative effort to hold an object close and thus achieve an enlargement.

During the low vision routine, determine the patient's response to the shorter working distance. It is important to remember that an ability to demonstrate the use of a spectacle magnifier in the consulting room does not necessarily translate into use in the patient's favorite armchair. Be alert to this possibility and warn patients of the importance of remembering to move objects into the appropriate position.

However, the main advantage of the spectacle magnifier is the improved field of view, when comparing this type of device with, for example, a spectacle mounted near telescope of the same magnification. An improved field of view may improve a patient's reading performance once the setback of working distance is overcome. As with all spectacle-mounted devices, the patient will have the use of both hands and if crouched over a table or having erected a reading stand, then he/she may be able to use a pen.

Another advantage is the acceptability of a spectacle, as many patients are expecting to be given 'strong glasses' so may adapt better than to, say, a telescopic system.

Note: if the patient has a spherical correction then this is easily compensated for within a singular spherical lens of the spectacle magnifier. That is, if the patient is a +12D aphake and requires a 4× spectacle magnifier (requiring a lens of 16D), then order a spectacle magnifier of 28D.

Hand magnifiers

There is an enormous variety of hand magnifiers available (Fig. 5.2a,b,c), with as much variety in cost and quality. Whether bought in a junk shop or found in amongst the old stamp collection, prescribed by a low vision practitioner, or found at an RNIB resource center, almost all patients who have suffered a visual

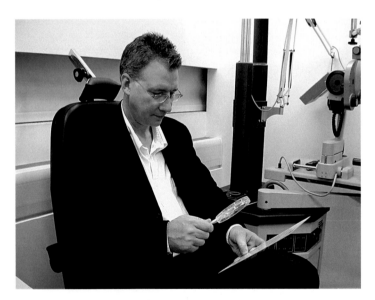

Figure 5.2(a) Hand magnifier in use

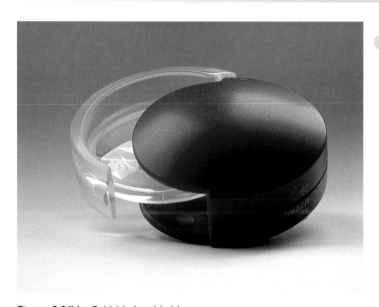

Figure 5.2(b) Foldable hand-held coupe

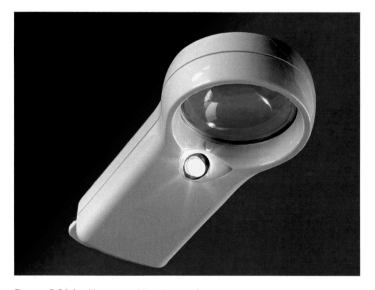

Figure 5.2(c) Illuminated hand magnifier

impairment will have tried using one in one form or another. Where available, it is important to ask the patient to bring their hand magnifier with them, even if they are finding it difficult to use. Often, increasing the addition in their currently unused reading spectacles may be sufficient to use the magnifier with greater efficiency.

Advantages include low cost, for many, and a wide range of magnification up to approximately 10–12×. They are portable and are more acceptable cosmetically to many elderly patients; generally, patients feel that using a hand magnifier in public is less likely to draw attention to them compared with using a spectacle-mounted telescope. The elderly often prefer this type of magnifier due to its ease of use and very many patients will acquire such an aid themselves before any formal visual assessment has been carried out.

Lens form may come as standard spherical or the more expensive aspheric which has all the usual advantages of asphericity (reduced aberrations, larger field of view for a given lens power). Illuminated versions are always available, most, if not all, are battery powered and come with tungsten or, increasingly, LED light sources. They may be used on their own, or in combination with the patient's current spectacles, distance or near.

One major disadvantage is that one hand is used in the process. The aid has to travel across the page and so the text is usually put on a flat surface if a book or a magazine is to be read. However, it is quite good for getting round corners and, as such, is good for 'spot checks' such as cooking instructions or dials on the washing machine where the patient has a variable head position and working distance. However, those with a hand tremor who have stiff joints or arthritic fingers will have difficulty in holding the aid and perhaps a spectacle magnifier or spectacle-mounted telescope here would be more suitable.

Effective magnification: what the patient actually achieves

The closer the aid is held to the object, the less will be the effective magnification. Maximum magnification is achieved when the magnifier is held at the focal length of the lens, which, for example, for a +10D magnifier will be 10 cm. However, at this distance the patient will experience **maximum** distortion and the **smallest** field of view. Therefore, it is easier for the patient if the magnifier is held slightly closer to the page. For this reason it is usually found that two different patients may have very different magnifications from the same hand magnifier.

Which spectacles?

Remember that the use of a hand magnifier is a dynamic system. Both pairs of spectacles, reading and distance, can be used but the position of the hand magnifier in relation to the object will vary, depending on the emergent vergence of the overall system.

A patient wearing their distance prescription will hold the hand magnifier closer to the focal point of the lens than will the patient wearing a near correction.

As the aid is a dynamic one, patients will tend to position the magnifier relative to the page such that the clearer image is found. So for distance spectacles, they will hold it further from the page. More typically, the aid is used in conjunction with a reading addition and so will be held closer to the page than the focal length of the lens.

Another useful point to remember when trying to decide whether a patient is achieving the desired magnification with their hand magnifier is to note the distance between the aid and the spectacles.

The hand magnifier and the reading addition in the spectacles combine to dictate the overall magnification. The equivalent power of the system is equal to the sum of the powers of the reading add (F_a) and the magnifier (F_m) minus the product of the two powers and the separation between them (z), thus:

$$\text{Equivalent power} = F_a + F_m - (zF_aF_m)$$

So in Fig. 5.1, if the spectacle add is +2.50D and the magnifier +20.00D, then if the separation is 5 cm (Fig. 5.3a) the equivalent power will be +20.00D (which is eight times the power the patient presented with). If z is zero (Fig. 5.3b) then

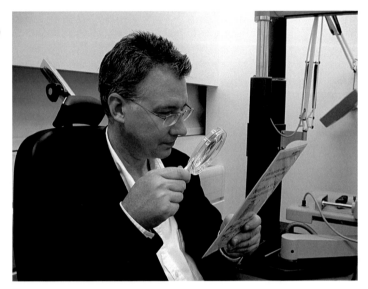

a

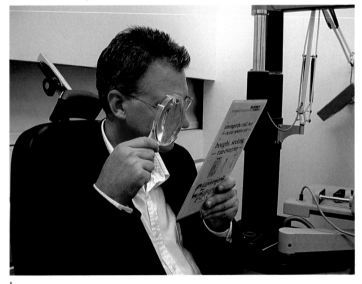

b

Figure 5.3(a) and (b) Use of a hand magnifier in conjunction with varifocals. The magnifier to spectacle distance influences the magnification

the equivalent power will be 22.50DS (nine times the starting value). Only when z gets larger (Fig. 5.2a) does the magnification reduce. So the maximum magnification and field of view is gained when the lens is held up against the addition, but then one in effect has a spectacle magnifier with the inconvenience of having to hold one of the components making this a non-viable alternative to strong spectacles.

It is very important to demonstrate clearly to the patient the use of a hand magnifier. The magnifier should be moved away from the object viewed until the image is found (usually when the aid is held just closer than its focal length from the object). Keeping this aid-to-object distance constant, the eye may then be moved closer to the magnifier to improve the field of view but bearing in mind the effect this distance has on the magnification achieved.

From a practical viewpoint, patients tend to like using these magnifiers due to their ease of use. But using a hand magnifier for great volumes of text is usually too much for most. The hand gets tired and the major complaint is that the aid has to be moved across the page all the time and thus keeping the text in focus can be hard work. This is even more an issue if a higher-powered magnifier is being used, as the field of view will be quite restrictive.

Lack of patience and an increase in frustration is usually the main complaint that patients will have when they return for a follow-up visit. As with all aids, the compromising reading position is often too much to overcome. Because of the rapid reduction in focal length with increasing power of the lens, high-powered hand magnifiers are rarely found as they rapidly convert into a form of stand magnifier (i.e. are held onto the viewing surface).

As a general rule, the authorities often found that for the elderly population, anything beyond a +20D (×6 Trade) hand magnifier gets too difficult to use. Younger users tend to have more patience and are often more adept.

Stand magnifiers

Reasons for changing to stand magnifiers from hand magnifiers include:

- Shaky hands.
- Higher magnification required—a wide range is available (Fig. 5.4a,b,c).

If, for example, the patient achieved a reasonable reading performance for the task with a 20DS hand magnifier, but found keeping it steady too awkward then start by demonstrating a stand magnifier of similar magnification. It may be useful to demonstrate a slightly lower magnification to begin with, for example here, a +16D stand magnifier, and then increase

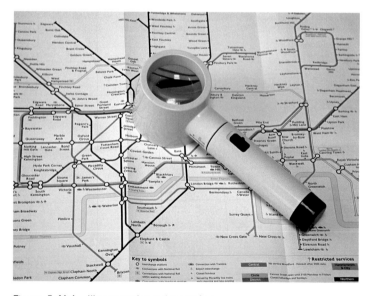

Figure 5.4(a) Illuminated stand magnifier

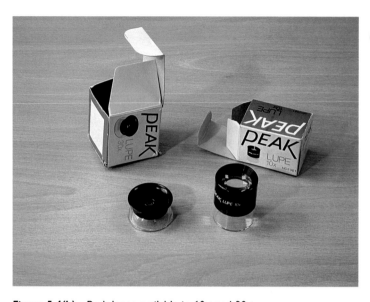

Figure 5.4(b) Peak lupes available in 10× and 30×

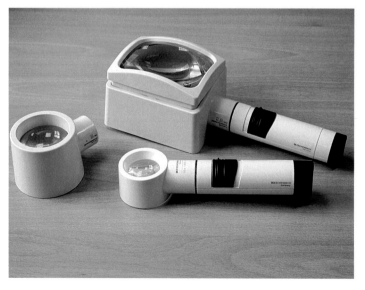

Figure 5.4(c) Range of illuminated stand magnifier

the level of magnification as the patient's reading performance improves.

Taking an initial step backwards is often useful as it is likely that the patient was using the previous hand magnifier within the focal length of the lens, so possibly not attaining its maximum magnification anyway.

Disadvantages

Stand magnifiers may be bulky and are generally not as portable as a similar powered hand magnifier. The patient must get as close to the lens as possible to achieve the maximal field of view, though this will also increase the accommodative demand or size of reading addition if a clear image is to be maintained (Fig. 5.5).

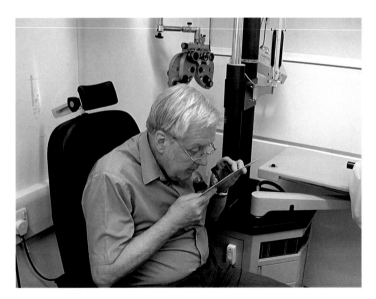

Figure 5.5 Stand magnifier in use—the closer the spectacle to magnifier distance, the higher the addition required

Other disadvantages include:

- Flat and firm surface needed.
- In the higher powers, the closer the patient gets to the page, the more important will be the inclusion of integral lighting, which will then increase the bulk and of course the cost.

Advantages

Hand tremor is a problem, then a stand magnifier is a good option. Due to the fixed working distance, text is kept in focus all the time and the patient can leave the device over the object and come back to it later. As a result, patients can use higher ranges of magnification with greater ease than a similar powered hand magnifier. They are hand-held stand magnifiers: not to be confused with a hand magnifier as they still have a fixed lens–object separation.

Larger stand magnifiers in the lower magnification range may come tilted, the idea here being that the patient may be able to get a pen underneath. Some do indeed manage this, but most prefer to use a thick black pen and a larger piece of paper.

Illuminated versions are available and some companies offer halogen illuminated systems within their range. Such magnifiers often have a rechargeable battery pack, which will require charging from the mains, or run directly from the mains, rendering the device less portable.

Most modern illuminated stand magnifiers are ordered with an LED light source (Fig. 5.6). This gives an intense blue-tinged light that offers good contrast for many ocular diseases but also has the very great advantage that the power usage is much less. The batteries will therefore last up to ten times longer, which is a significant advantage for many users.

Lens–object separation

If the lens of the stand magnifier is set at f_1 from the object (the anterior focal length) then the emergent rays (vergence) are parallel. Thus, to the patient's eye, the image of the object would appear to be set at infinity. In order to focus this image, the

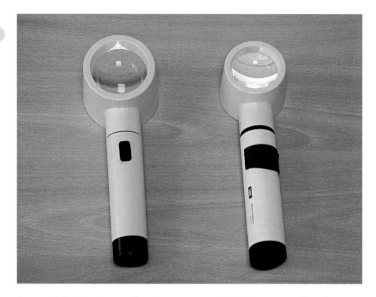

Figure 5.6 Stand magnifier fitted with an LED light source (right)

patient will need to wear their distance correction and all accommodative effort is relaxed.

Conversely, if the lens-to-object distance is less than the focal length of the lens, then the emergent rays are divergent and the patient will need either to accommodate or use their reading spectacles to focus the image. It is often of importance, therefore, for the patient to keep any old spectacles as it may mean that they will be able to get optimum efficiency from the aid prescribed.

There are a few stand magnifiers that will have the facility to adjust the lens–object separation. Here, the minute changes in lens–object separation can be made to the high-powered stand magnifier to allow for changes in the emergent vergence, thus adjusting the focus for the patient.

If the lens is set at the focal length from the page such that light leaving the lens is parallel, then maximum magnification is achieved but at the expense of image quality. There will be significant aberration, particularly chromatic, which will degrade the image quality. For this reason, the vast majority of modern stand magnifiers are set closer to the page than the focal length

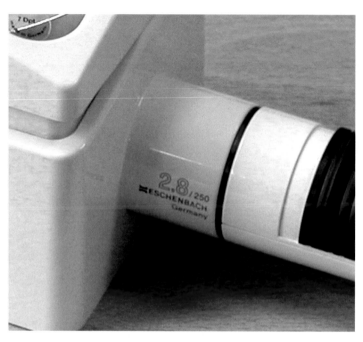

Figure 5.7 Eschenbach series stand magnifiers indicating magnification (2.8) and working distance (250 mm)

of the lens so requiring accommodation or a reading add to view the image clearly. Many aids, such as the Eschenbach series shown in Fig. 5.7, carry a number representing the recommended working distance for the aid (in the example shown, 250 mm) when used with a standard (usually +2.50D) addition. If a patient is failing to get on with a stand magnifier, observe them using it. If they have to lift the aid off the task surface in order to gain a clear view then they have an inappropriate addition that will need increasing or they may have insufficient accommodation (as, perhaps, may happen with a visually impaired diabetic patient approaching presbyopia).

If, on the other hand, a patient is coping well with the image quality but finds the field of view achieved through the stand magnifier limiting, then moving their eye closer to the aid may improve the field of view but render the image out of focus.

In this case, a useful approach would be to increase the reading addition of the spectacles the patient is using. Often it is a matter of small incremental steps over the existing addition until a clarity is reached with which the patient is happy.

Field of view

The field of view of the image will vary, depending on the distance the eye is from the magnifier lens.

Is it at f_1 or within f_1?

Knowledge of the lens–object distance is important before demonstrating a new aid to a patient. There are a number of ways that this can be done:

Using a distant light source

Hold the stand magnifier on a page under a highly placed ceiling light (the nearer to infinity the better). If the lens is set at f_1 then the light will focus to a near-point source on a piece of paper placed underneath the magnifier on the floor/table. If it is set within f_1 then lifting the magnifier off the page will be necessary to gain the same point image.

Measure the lens–object separation

From a more practical level, measure the distance that the lens is set from the page, or object. If a 20D stand magnifier is set at f_1, then the lens–object separation will be 5 cm. If it is set within f_1 then it will be less than 5 cm. (Usually just over 4 cm in this example.) However, remember that these are thick lenses so the measurement will be an approximation. If the distance were significantly less than 5 cm (which it may not be), it would be safe to conclude that the lens is set within f_1. This simple technique also allows a practitioner to estimate the emergent vergence from the aid.

Look through it

Look through the stand magnifier at the image, say a line of text. Then lift the aid off the page. If the image goes immediately out of focus, then it was at f_1. If it remains in focus for a small distance, then the reverse applies.

By positioning the lens closer to the page than f_1, the field of view is better and there is less distortion of the image. However, the effective magnification will be less. Those magnifiers which are set at or as near as possible to f_1 will have the higher magnification for a given lens power but a comparably lesser field of view. To minimize the distortion then more expensive aspheric lenses tend to be used.

A note on magnification

Magnification might be thought of as the ratio of the angle of subtense at the retina of an object and the increased angle when it is magnified. This may be achieved in several ways. Relative size magnification is the increase in an angle of subtense resulting from simply making something larger. This is achieved by, for example, large-print books or buying a large-screen television.

Most simple aids (spectacle, hand and stand magnifiers) exploit relative distance magnification in that they allow an object to be seen at a closer distance and therefore subtend a larger angle at the retina and thus be seen as larger.

Telescopes allow an image even in the far distance to be seen as larger by exploiting angular magnification. A sequence of lenses increases the angle of subtense of incoming light while the object distance remains constant.

For the purposes of classification and ordering, magnifiers tend to be calibrated in terms of magnification. This relies on some formulation allowing a magnification value to be derived from knowing the dioptric value of the lens in the aid.

If one assumes an object Q to be placed at the anterior focal plane of the lens before an emmetropic eye, then the image formed Q′ will be formed at infinity (Fig. 5.8). If one then looks at the situation before the lens was in place (Fig. 5.9) then the magnification M will be the ratio of the two angles of subtense, u'/u. The two angles may be defined in terms of the triangles they

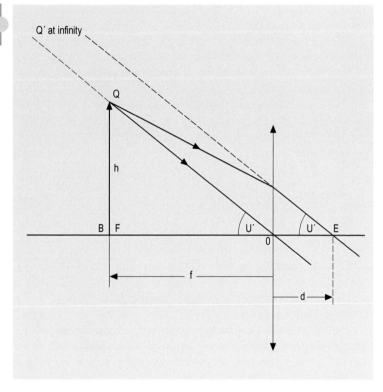

Figure 5.8 Image formed by an object Q placed at the anterior focal plane of a lens

are within, such that $u = -h/p$ and $u' = -h/f$. If the values are now put in to replace the angles in $M = u'/u$, then one is left with $M = -pF$. If one then assumes p to be -25 cm (the least distance of distinct vision) then one is left with the formula:

$$M = F/4$$

This is called the nominal magnification formula, but is based on several assumptions as outlined and also does not really

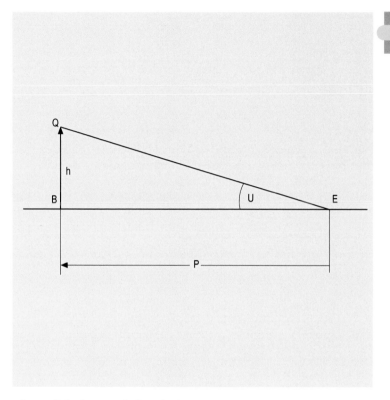

Figure 5.9 Situation before the lens was in place

represent how an aid might be used. More typically, an object will be held within the anterior focal plane of the lens such that an image is formed closer than infinity (see Fig. 5.10). If one now assumes that the object is placed close enough so that the image is formed at the anterior focal plane of the lens, say −25 cm for consistency, then algebraic derivation based on Fig. 5.9 will lead to the formula:

$$M = F/4 + 1$$

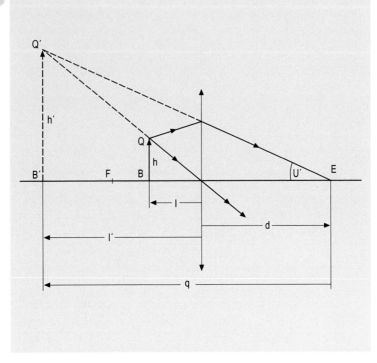

Figure 5.10 Image formed closer than infinity

In order to arrive at this, the value *d* representing the lens-to-eye distance must be assumed to be zero and the image-to-eye distance *q* must equal *p* in the unaided eye (which is −25 cm). This so-called trade magnification formula is the one most manufacturers subscribe to and it must be emphasized that it is most useful merely in comparing one aid with another and for categorizing aids. It often differs wildly from the actual magnification a patient will achieve in real life, which will depend on where they hold the lens and the original size of the image screen.

Telescopes

There are two designs of refractive telescope: Galilean and astronomical (or Keplerian). Both are afocal in design, i.e. they can be used to view objects at infinity.

Galilean telescope (Fig. 5.11)

The eyepiece is negative, and the objective is a positive lens. In an afocal telescope of this design, the separation

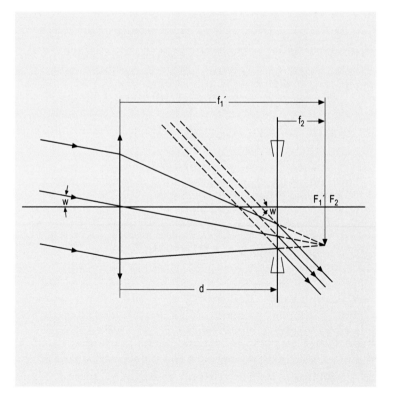

Figure 5.11 Galilean telescope

between the two lenses is the difference between their two focal lengths.

The resultant magnification in the telescope is positive, indicating that the image is erect.

$$M = -\frac{F_e}{F_o}$$

Galilean designs are limited to ×3 for distance viewing. The lack of a prism system will also make them more lightweight, and thus more appropriate for modification to be used for near vision magnification.

Astronomical (Keplerian) telescope (Fig. 5.12)

Here, both the eyepiece and objective lenses are convex and the image from this system will be inverted, indicated by a negative sign in the previous equation. Thus, a prism erecting system is incorporated into the system to re-erect the image.

The length of the telescope will be the sum of the focal lengths of the eyepiece and objective. Thus, astronomical designs are longer. The incorporation of the prism erecting system adds to the weight and bulk.

Although the Galilean telescopes are smaller and more compact units than their astronomical counterparts, the astronomical forms have effectively a better field of view and the image quality is superior (see later).

Compound lens systems

The eyepiece lens in both systems will be the more powerful of the two lenses. In many distance Galilean and most astronomical designs, a compound lens system may be used as either the eyepiece or objective (most likely the eyepiece lens). This means that there may be more than one lens cemented

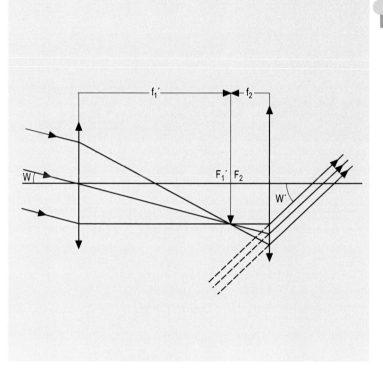

Figure 5.12 Astronomical telescope

to another, thus increasing the power of the overall
eyepiece or objective unit and keeping aberrations
comparatively low. In low vision aids, the power of these
lenses needs to be quite high, and thus they will have
appropriate design and coatings to improve overall optical
quality. It is important to remember, however, that the
number of lenses within the system will have an effect
of overall loss of brightness, and will also have the
additional disadvantage of making them heavier.

Other basic principles of afocal telescopes

Exit and entrance pupils

All rays entering a telescope through the objective lens, or entrance pupil, will leave through the exit pupil and then enter the eye through the patient's (entrance) pupil. The exit pupil of the telescope is the image of the objective lens as seen from the eyepiece side. In the Galilean system the exit pupil appears within, or internal to, the telescope system and with an astronomical design it appears between our eye and the eyepiece. In the latter design it is also much smaller in size. This is primarily due to the degree of magnification of the system and the size of the objective lens.

$$\text{Exit pupil diameter} = \frac{\text{objective lens diameter}}{\text{telescope magnification}}$$

The above equation can be used to estimate the telescope's magnification. The objective lens diameter is usually straightforward to measure. Furthermore, some devices have the size of the objective printed on the side of the casing. The exit pupil of an astronomical telescope is also simple to measure, although less so with the Galilean system, as it is internal.

Markings: what do they mean?

Many distance telescopes will have markings, for example:

8 × 20 LVA 7.5°

where

8×	the magnification
20	the diameter of the objective lens in mm.
7.5°	the field of view

'Extra short focus' means that the basic telescope design can be modified to view an object at a closer working distance.

Field of view

The field of view increases with the diameter of the objective. If the exit pupil of the telescope is placed as close as possible to the entrance pupil of the eye, then the field of view is maximized. This is clearly easier with the astronomical system, where the exit pupil is between the eyepiece lens and the patient's pupil. In the case of a Galilean system, the exit pupil can be several millimeters away and thus the overall field of view is less than stated by the manufacturer. In both cases, if the patient is going to use the telescope held against their spectacle lens, then the field of view will decrease again, according to the spectacle lens BVD (back vertex distance).

In practice: using a telescope as a low vision aid

Both the astronomical and Galilean telescope designs are afocal: they will focus infinitely distant objects only. In reality, when a telescope is to be used as a low vision aid, the majority of objects that a patient needs to be able to view will not be at infinity. Secondly, eyes tend not to be emmetropic and for the most part, the basic afocal design will require modification. Any modification will ultimately have an effect on the overall resultant magnification.

Vergence amplification

Incident vergence is amplified, or magnified, when it passes through a telescope system. This means that incident vergence from a near object will be magnified at the point it enters the eye through the entrance pupil.

An *approximate* formula is:

Emergent vergence = (Magnification)^2 × Incident vergence

Example 1

A 6× distance monocular is used to view a train indicator board at a distance of 3 m:

$$\text{Emergent vergence} = (6)^2 \times 0.3D$$
$$= 10.8D$$

When an emmetropic or corrected eye is used to view an object at 3 m, a negligible amount of accommodative effort (0.3D) is necessary. However, once the incident vergence of 0.3D is amplified through the telescope, the emergent vergence entering the eye will be almost 11D. Thus, the patient will need to accommodate by that amount the focus of the image on the retina. This is clearly unacceptable.

Example 2

An 8× afocal distance monocular is used to view an object at 25 cm:

$$\text{Emergent vergence} = (8)^2 \times 4D$$
$$= 256D$$

To view an object at 25 cm, either 4D of accommodation is necessary, or an appropriate presbyopic correction (+4.00D addition in a completely presbyopic eye). According to the above equation, however, when using an afocal telescope to view the same object, we would need an impossible accommodative effort of 256D.

Effect of changing the telescope length

The optical ray path will alter as soon as the separation between the eyepiece and objective lenses is increased or decreased. There are two major purposes for doing this:

1. To compensate for the patient's refractive error.
2. To view a finite object, usually intermediate or near.

Many telescopes will therefore have variable focus.

Correcting for ametropia

An afocal telescope can be simply cemented or clipped onto the front surface of the patient's spectacles. However, this may not be altogether very practical (or attractive), so the easiest way to compensate for ametropia is to change the length of the tube, i.e. increase or decrease the separation between the eyepiece and the objective lenses.

- A myope shortens the tube length: emergent vergence from the exit pupil is thus diverged to the degree necessary to compensate for the myopia.
- A hypermetrope will lengthen the tube length to create a convergent light beam.

This will hold true for moderate degrees of ametropia only. Higher degrees of refractive error cannot be corrected in this way due to the restrictions in the size of altering the tube lengths.

Worked example

Galilean telescope:

F_e	−40D
F_o	+20D
$M = -F_e/F_o =$	2×

Tube length = $f_o' + f_e'$ = 50 + (−25) = 25 mm

If a −5D myope were to use the telescope and refocus to compensate for ammetropia, he will theoretically 'borrow' 5D from the −40D eyepiece, leaving it as a −35D eyepiece lens:

F_e	−35D
F_o	+20D
$M =$	1.75×
Tube length:	21.4 mm

If the above example is used again for an astronomical telescope, the amount of effective magnification will also change.

A myope will achieve more magnification from using an astronomical telescope compared to a Galilean design offering the same magnification. The reverse is true for a hypermetrope, i.e. the hypermetrope will achieve more magnification from a Galilean design, but less if using an astronomical design.

Viewing an object closer than infinity

Most astronomical distance telescopes may be focused to a fairly close distance. This can be achieved by extending the tube length.

'Extra-short focus'

This is often printed on the side of a monocular telescope. By increasing the distance between the eyepiece and the objective lenses, the incident vergence from the near placed object (e.g. a vergence of −4D if the object is placed at 25 cm, −2D if placed at 50 cm) can be corrected so that it enters the telescope parallel. Magnification will alter also, becoming greater. This facility tends to be used more for notice boards than for actual reading text from a book or a page. Viewing an object closer than 25 cm will place a practical limitation on the extension of the telescope.

Adding an end cap

Another way of correcting for viewing a near object would be to add an **end-cap** to the objective lens. This end-cap, which will be a lens of the dioptric equivalent to the emergent vergence (e.g. a +4D lens if viewing at 25 cm, a +10D lens if viewing at 10 cm, etc.), would neutralize the incident vergence entering the telescope system. Thus, light passing through the system will be again parallel and there will be no vergence amplification effect.

The power of the end-cap will have an effect on the overall magnification of the system. The overall magnification will be the product of the magnification provided by both the objective and the reading cap.

Viewing an object at $12\frac{1}{2}$ cm will require a +8.00D end-cap, which will give an extra ×2 magnification ($M = F/4$; thus, $8/4 = 2$).

If this is placed over the objective of a ×4 monocular, then the overall magnification effect will be (×4) × (×2) = ×8.

An important point here is that if we compare the working distance of the above telescope with a spectacle magnifier of the same effective magnification (4× = 32D), then there is a notable difference in the working distance. The focal length (and thus the working distance) of the latter will be shorter, around 3 cm only.

If an end-cap is used, then the object will need to be placed at the focal length of this lens. This will be quite restrictive in use as a low vision aid, as the patient will need to be able to use the device at a number of different distances.

Adding a lens to the eyepiece

This is a useful way to compensate for any refractive error that the patient may have, especially if the patient has a significant cyl. Theoretically, a situation could also arise whereby the power of the spectacle lens could be sufficient to compensate for any amplified vergence as it leaves the exit pupil of the system. However, given that the power of the spectacle lens would often be high, this becomes an impractical solution. Instead, one might:

● Hold the telescope/binoculars up to the spectacles.
● Use spectacle clip telescopes.
● Cement the telescopes (binocular/monocular) to the front surface of the spectacle lens.

There will be no additional effect on the telescopic magnification as the vergence of the light entering the patient's pupil from the telescope is unchanged, and parallel as before. However, if the exit pupil of the telescope is placed further away from the entrance pupil of the eye, the overall effect will be additionally to reduce the patient's field of view.

Using a near telescope as a low vision aid

Following on from the previous discussions, the afocal telescope is modified to become a near vision (focal) telescope by either:

1. Increasing the separation between the eyepiece and objective lenses, or
2. Adding more plus to the objective lens, either by incorporating the power into the objective lens itself or by the addition of the end-cap. The working distance of the near telescope will be the anterior focal point of the additional plus.

Cyl correction

Possibly, another slight advantage is that if the patient has a significant cylindrical correction, then this can be incorporated into the spectacle lens that the telescope is cemented onto. As with spectacle magnifiers, there are some designs of telescopes that can be interchanged by cementing a carrier onto the front surface of the patient's spectacle lens. This is useful if the patient needs two different telescopes, or equally important if the VA alters.

Advantages and disadvantages of telescopes

Distance telescopes

Telescopes tend to be a more expensive type of device. They are also heavy, bulky and difficult to get used to. Thus, training may be necessary in many cases. Patients may also feel conspicuous especially when using one in public. But most of all, the field of view is very restricted indeed; most distance telescopes, for example, have approximately a 7° field.

The major advantage for using a distance telescope is that for many, it is the only practical method of magnification for distance viewing. The only other way to increase the retinal image size is to walk closer to the object. But for practical purposes, this may not often be possible. However, once the patient is able to use a device successfully, lifestyle is often transformed, most especially in those patients who lead mobile lives.

Distance telescopes may be:

- Hand-held (monoculars or binoculars).
- Spectacle mounted (monoculars or binoculars).
- Head-borne sets (binocular).

Note: higher powered telescopes are bulkier and heavier; therefore, the latter two are limited to lower powers only, generally to about 3×.

Near telescopes

The major advantage of a near vision telescope is the increased working distance compared to the spectacle magnifier offering the same magnification. We often directly compare and contrast these two aids as they are (for the most part) both spectacle mounted.

If a patient requests a hands-free option after trying out a hand or stand magnifier, then one would generally try out the spectacle magnifier first. If the patient then has difficulty adapting to the close working distance a telescope can be tried as an alternative.

The major advantage for having a near vision spectacle-mounted telescope is resultant increase in working distance. The rest are obviously a disadvantage: there is an increased weight problem, cosmetically they may be unacceptable, they are significantly more costly and the field of view is poor.

Range of magnifications available for near

Binocularly, Keeler long-tube telescopes go up to 5×. The tubes are angled inwards to compensate for the required convergence. Beyond this, more magnification is impossible binocularly due to the restriction of the tube convergence. Monocularly, 8x would currently appear to be the limit. Anything higher than this, and then the difference in working distance between the telescope and the spectacle magnifier becomes less and thus not worthwhile. Examples of near telescopes include:

- Keeler's GWide Vu Magnifier (LVA 22) (Fig. 5.13):
  a. Up to 8× monocularly, 3× binocularly.
  b. Wider field, but shorter working distance up to 14 cm.
- Keeler's Read–Write magnifier (LVA 21):
  a. Up to 8× monocularly, 5× binocularly.
  b. *Longer tube, less field of view but improved working distance of up to 15 cm.*
- Eschenbach's Galilean binocular systems for near (up to 4×).

Distance telescopes and binoculars

Hand-held telescopes are usually for distance use and may be easily obtained up to 10× (12× and 15× are available although are less frequently used). Binoculars are easily obtained up to 12× or more. (Typically, 4×, 6× and 8× are most commonly used).

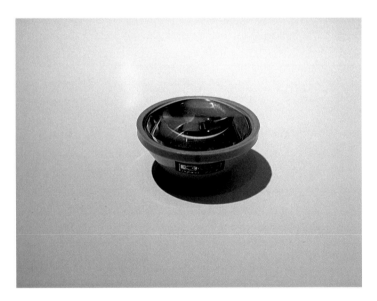

Figure 5.13   A fixed focus near Galilean telescope

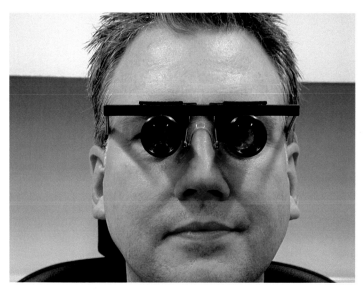

Figure 5.14 Distance telescope system tried for television use

Spectacle mounted telescope systems may be tried for, for example, television viewing (Fig. 5.14).

Prescribing

As astronomical telescopes are significantly heavier they tend not to be spectacle mounted. However, in the Galilean designs there are the popular ×3 Eschenbach binoculars, which may be used for static distance viewing, such as in a classroom, or watching TV.

Hand-held telescopes are useful for viewing stable static objects in the distance for a short period, e.g. train notice boards, shop signs, etc. It is a myth that they are used successfully for moving targets such as checking the number of moving buses, although, after training, they may occasionally be used for this purpose.

Identification of telescope design (Table 5.2)

Galilean telescopes are used mainly for viewing near objects. The majority of astronomical types are used for distance.

Table 5.2 Identification of telescope design

Method of identification	Galilean	Astronomical
Feeling the eyepiece	Concave It may be obvious in simple near telescope systems which are made up of two lenses but often the eyepiece may be made up of a compound lens system, with even a plano or convex front vertex power	Convex Often not easy to determine by 'feel' alone so this method has its drawbacks
Size	Smaller, shorter	Longer tube length, heavier due to prism incorporation
Distance or near?	Tend to be for near viewing Most fixed focus near telescopes will be Galilean (e.g. Keeler, Rayner, Stigmat).	Tend to be for distance Most, if not all, are variable focus
Variable focus?	There are some low-power distance telescopes and binoculars, usually with a small degree of variable focus (Eschenbach binoculars tend to be of Galilean design)	There are one/two manufactured which are spectacle mounted (clip or cemented) of astronomical design
Power	Limited to ×3 max. for distance	Tend to be limited to ×2–×4 when spec-mounted, otherwise they get too large and heavy, requiring them to be hand-held

	For near will go as high as 8× monocularly, 5× binocularly	For distance viewing will go as high as 15×, although 6× and 8× (both monoc. and binoc.) are most popular
Prism	Not integrated as erect image	By looking down the wrong end, the prism correcting system may be viewed
Position of the exit pupil*	Internal By placing a finger at the objective lens and looking at it through the eyepiece. Does it look as though it is inside the tube?	External Hold up the telescope but slightly away from you. If the image of the exit pupil appears in front of the eyepiece, then the telescope is astronomical. The exit pupil is very small. If a finger is placed at the end of the tube now, it can barely be seen
Size of the exit pupil*	Outer edge of exit pupil not all visible	Whole of exit pupil visible in one position of view
The positive eyepiece means that the outline of the objective lens when viewed through the eyepiece will move 'against' when the viewer holds the aid still and wobbles their head	With movement	Against movement

*The exit pupil represents the image of the entrance pupil

Summary

HAND MAGNIFIERS

Advantages	Disadvantages
Inexpensive (esp. non-aspheric)	Rely on steady hand/one hand used up
Socially acceptable	
May be illuminated	Non-aspheric may have poorer image quality
Portable	Effective mag often less (held within f_1)
Allow writing or tool use	Often needs to be explained to patient

STAND MAGNIFIERS

Advantages	Disadvantages
High mag. possible (e.g. 30×)	Poor field of view at high magnifier
May be illuminated	May be bulky
Lower mag. may tilt for writing	May require near correction adjustments
Steady for shaky hands	
High mag. may be adjustable for accommodation/vergence difficulties	

SPECTACLE MAGNIFIERS

Advantages	Disadvantages
Good field of view	Short working distance
Wide range of appliances	Binocularity/convergence problems
Cosmetically/psychologically acceptable	
Adaptable (coats, tints, etc.)	
Hands free	

TELESCOPES

Advantages	Disadvantages
Distance or near	Expensive
Binocular or monocular	Poor cosmesis
Increased working distance	Heavy
Variable focus	Training required
May be spectacle mounted (hands free)	Magnification of body movement
	Poor field of view

6
Electronic magnification

The use of a closed-circuit television (CCTV) system as an aid for low visual acuity was suggested in 1959 after initial work by Genensky et al.[70] This was later developed by Genensky and coworkers in the 1970s.[71,72]

The concept of using a CCTV as a low vision aid has, therefore, been a reality for some time. Despite the advantages of an enhanced image and significantly more magnification than optical devices, the high cost and lack of portability has previously limited their use to the workplace or schoolroom where funding may be obtained from central government. Thus, in the home, many optical aids have been, by default, more acceptable due to relatively low cost and portability for most patients.

CCTVs for all

The advancements in information technology and quality of equipment now readily available have significantly widened the use of electronic magnification.[73] All age groups are now regular computer users and as relative costs reduce and portability improve, it is predicted that domestic use will become commonplace. In time the elderly will turn to electronic magnification as a principal method of magnification. It would therefore be unwise for a low vision practitioner to limit his or her consultations to the use of optical devices. Harvey[74] argued that the use of electronic magnification should now become a regular feature of low vision consultations within all age groups.

Real image magnification

With optical magnification the image is viewed at or within the lens-to-object working distance, i.e. the focal length of the plus lens. This will be eventually limited at a level of magnification that is impractical to use due to the physical constraints of the short working distance.

Real image magnification, however, can be electronically produced onto a display screen or monitor and the magnification

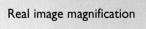

so produced is significantly higher than that of optical devices. Whereas optical magnification is limited to approximately 30× (working distance 3.33 cm), the magnification produced on the screen may be as much as 40–60×. The limitations to magnification that has been electronically produced will be as a result of the quality of the technology and the size of the screen.

The conventional CCTV

The CCTV is the most commonly recognized electronic magnification system. A video camera with integral zoom system is set above a movable *XY* table. This captures an image of the object from the *XY* table that is then displayed 'live' onto the monitor in front of the patient, typically at eye level.

Features regularly incorporated within systems may include:

- Brightness adjustment.
- Contrast enhancement.
- Color or monochrome.
- Image reversal.
- Underlining or highlighting.
- Text isolation: areas of unwanted script or isolating single lines.

It is also now possible to combine a desktop computer with a CCTV system; dual presentation is managed on a split screen.

Advantages of CCTV systems

- Wide range of magnification, up to 40–60×, is often achievable, which is useful for those who may have a progressive loss of acuity.
- Systems can permit a rapid change in magnification without loss of focus.
- A wide range of uses, from the school/office to the home.
- Less fatigue: use of the CCTV maintains a binocular view, and eliminates problems of convergence and the uncomfortable reading posture that is often problematic with high-level

optical magnification. With this advantage, sustained reading tasks may be possible, although success will rest with the acuity reserve as discussed in previous sections.

- Acceptable cosmosis.
- Image reversal: most patients utilize the image reversal capabilities of the systems to produce white text on a black background. The reduction in light scatter within the eye is useful to many who have media opacities or who have photosensitivity.
- Contrast enhancement: for patients with low contrast sensitivity. Increases the potential for success by improving contrast reserve.
- Mechanisms now exist that can capture distant or intermediate objects which can be presented on the display screen.

Field of view

The field of view of any system is dependent on screen size and magnification. Increasing the screen size will have the advantage of producing a greater field of view although this may have the disadvantage of requiring larger and heavier equipment.

With optical magnification, the closer the patient is to the plus lens, the greater will be the field of view, and the greater the number of characters visible. However, with a CCTV system, the field of view is not influenced by eye–monitor distance, unless the patient is very close to the monitor, when the reverse becomes true. By moving closer to the screen, there will come a point at which the size of the monitor will extend beyond the patient's own field of view and the patient will need to turn his or her head to view the object viewed on the screen.

Using relative distance magnification and steady eye strategy

Most patients will often sit at eye level to the monitor and at a comfortable viewing distance. Presbyopic patients may prefer a reading addition. However, as previously suggested, some patients may sit much closer, gaining additional relative

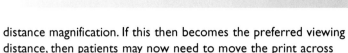
distance magnification. If this then becomes the preferred viewing distance, then patients may now need to move the print across their field of view and use a steady eye strategy.

Steady eye strategy is easier with the CCTV system than with optical devices. Text is easily moved through the preferred retinal locus (PRL) by using the XY table or mouse. Patients with significant restriction of the visual field often prefer this method.

Portable systems

TV readers

Portable systems are now available, which expands the use of the CCTV system within the home environment. The first to appear on the market were the 'TV readers' which used the patient's own television as the display screen. The television is simply connected up to the camera set within a 'mouse' that fits into the patient's hand. The mouse is then moved over the printed text or object and the image is displayed on the television screen (see Fig. 6.1a and b).

Systems are available in both color and monochrome. Most include options for a small range of magnifications, and reverse polarity is usually common to all. Additional magnification may be gained by using a larger television screen.

Video magnifiers

These are essentially portable CCTV systems, with rechargeable battery packs capable of sustaining up to 4 hours of usage. The single unit incorporates both the display screen and the camera and is placed over the object at a fixed distance (Fig. 6.2a and b). Features include a singular or small range of magnification, brightness and contrast enhancement, and monochrome or color models are available. Most are lighter in weight than a laptop computer and some are small enough to put in a pocket or handbag.

Many have additional features that will allow them to be connected up to the patient's television at home, allowing for additional magnification or an alternative viewing position.

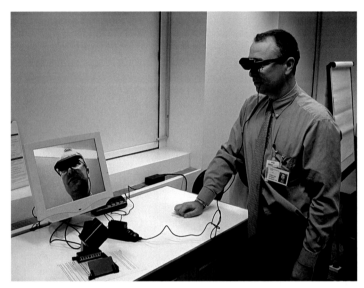

a

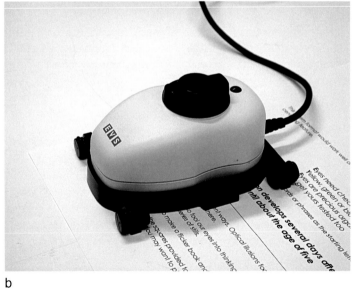

b

Figure 6.1(a) and (b) A portable TV reader in use

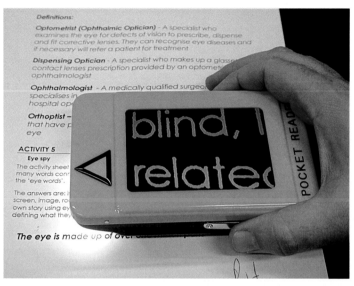

a

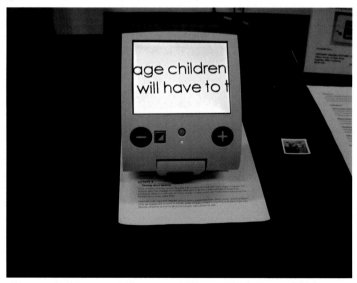

b

Figure 6.2(a) and (b)   Video magnifiers

Head-mounted displays

Within the last decade there has been a significant advance in the development of head-mounted systems (Fig. 6.3). These have been marketed as revolutionary in the field of low vision.

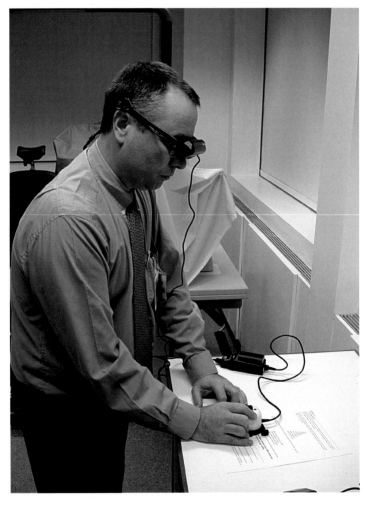

Figure 6.3 A head-mounted display in use

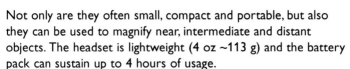

Not only are they often small, compact and portable, but also they can be used to magnify near, intermediate and distant objects. The headset is lightweight (4 oz ~113 g) and the battery pack can sustain up to 4 hours of usage.

The basic principles of these systems are similar to those of the conventional CCTV; the miniature camera, usually hand held or set within a mouse, is connected to a high-quality liquid crystal display (LCD) screen set in front of the patient's eyes. A variety of systems are now in existence and magnification is variable up to 25× approximately.

Some have the additional feature that they may be placed within a docking stand connected in a display unit allowing for additional magnification up to 40–50×.

7

Additional strategies and non-optical methods for improving visual performance

In previous chapters, relative distance magnification is the main strategy for improving visual performance, which low vision practitioners use. However, there are a number of alternative approaches to aid visually impaired patients in the environment, which the practitioner may discuss within the consulting room.

Relative size magnification

The retinal image size can be simply increased by increasing the size of the object:

$$\text{Magnification} = \frac{\text{new object size}}{\text{old object size}}$$

The RNIB produce a number of catalogs that are available for both the practitioner and the patient, which give examples of larger items. These include:

- Large print books, newspapers and magazines.
- Large button telephones (Fig. 7.1a).
- Watches and clocks.
- Games for adults and children (Fig. 7.1b,c).
- Some household items and kitchen equipment.

Using large print

Standard print size for most printed material is produced in N10–N12. (Many books produced for small children may be produced in larger print.) Large print books and newspapers are typically N18–N24, which is approximately 2–2½× larger than standard print. Equally important are the spacing between lines and the typeface chosen and, of course, the level of contrast used. These factors will add to the cost of publication.

Large print books are popular with elderly patients as a method of magnification as it is both cosmetically acceptable and aids normal reading posture (Fig. 7.2). Patients may still read with the book 'on the lap' and view the book binocularly. No special training or advice is necessary when this method is chosen and

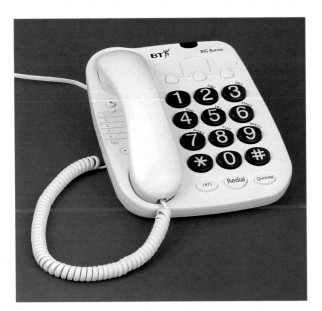

a

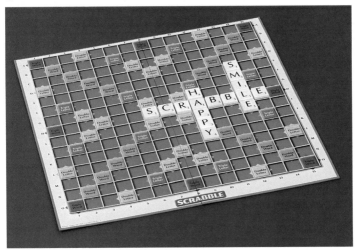

b

Figure 7.1 (a) Big button telephone; (b) and (c) Large print Scrabble

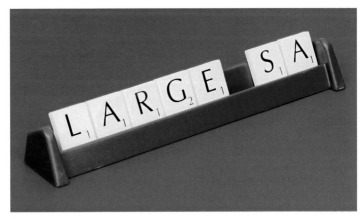

c

Figure 7.1 cont'd

often the patient will have already used some form of large print
before they have chosen to attend a low vision consultation.

With a further reduction in visual acuity, patients with
a progressive loss may need to use low vision aids to view large
print publications, therefore combining both methods of
magnification.

To produce 2½ magnification in large print, the book or paper
itself will increase in size. Often this brings additional problems.
Books become larger and bulkier and often difficult to produce.
Thinner paper can be used, but patients have regularly
complained that the print from the underlying pages becomes
visible and hence either bothersome or impossible to use.
Abridged versions of novels are, by rights of publication, are often
unacceptable.

'Big print'

Launched in 1992, 'Big Print' is the only British weekly newspaper
that is published with bold text in double the normal type size.
It promotes itself as a 'broad spectrum newspaper with no
political bias' and aims to cater for most tastes. It comprises
national and international news coverage, provided by the
country's leading news agencies. In addition, there is sports

Figure 7.2 Large print dictionary

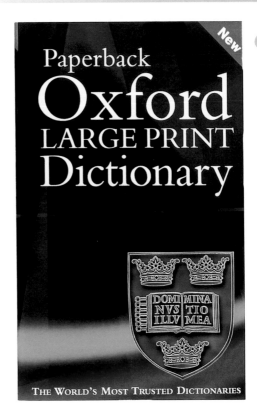

Paperback
Oxford
LARGE PRINT
Dictionary

THE WORLD'S MOST TRUSTED DICTIONARIES

coverage and leisure reading, including a horoscope, crossword, word puzzles and large print book reviews, together with a comprehensive listing of radio and television programs for the following week. The newspaper has a readership of around 18,000 and has the marketing support of the RNIB.

Large print documents such as bus maps and the London Tube map are also available (Figs. 7.3 and 7.4). Children often benefit from enlarging schoolwork or printed text larger. Most photocopiers can do this without a significant loss of contrast or quality.

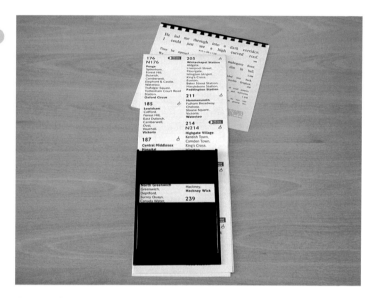

Figure 7.3 Large print address sheet under a typoscope

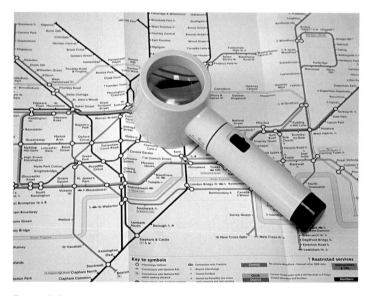

Figure 7.4 Large print tube map

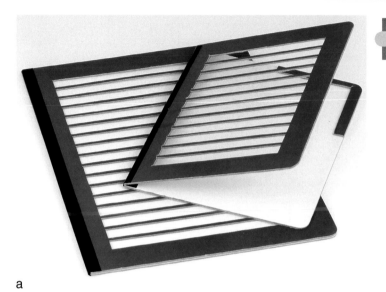

a

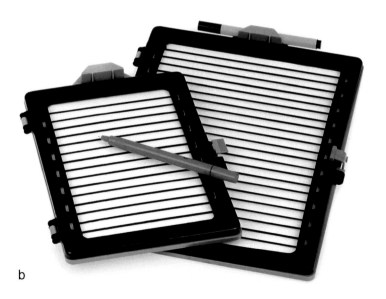

b

Figure 7.5(a) and (b) Writing frames

The RNIB also produce a selection of thick-lined stationery and a writing grid which can be used to write documents or letters (Fig. 7.5).

Full listings of large-print publications and stationery may be obtained from the RNIB.

Management of photophobia and glare sensitivity

Photophobia and glare sensitivity are commonly encountered visual impairments. Exposure to different types of light and lighting can be, for many, uncomfortable or even painful. This will have functional implication for a number of patients. For example:

- The patient may suffer a significantly reduced vision/visual acuity.
- Changes may be necessary within the home or work environment.
- Sunglasses, filters or visors may be necessary.
- Task lighting will need to be adapted to suit the individual.

Although not a criterion for certification (i.e. sight impaired/ seriously sight impaired), there is now a section included in the CVI (2003) that the consultant ophthalmologist will complete, which will indicate whether the patient's vision is known to vary markedly under different light levels.[11,14]

Examples of some conditions or circumstances that may give rise to photophobia or glare sensitivity[75] include:

- Corneal pathologies, including dystrophies, abrasion or trauma.
- Contact lens problems.
- Following refractive surgery.
- Uveitis.
- Cataract.

- Retinitis pigmentosa.
- Albinism.
- Diabetic retinopathy.
- Macular degeneration.
- Macular dystrophy.
- Rod cone dystrophy.
- Glaucoma.
- CNS disorders such as meningitis.
- Botulism.
- Mercury poisoning.
- Rabies.
- Drug-induced, e.g. quinine, atropine, tetracycline.
- Migraine.
- Sunburn.

Photophobia

The term photophobia is used widely by practitioners to describe any sensitivity to light. Strictly speaking, true photophobia is a symptom caused by a pathology affecting the corneal sensory nerve endings, which includes pain, excessive tearing and blepharospasm. For example, a corneal pathology such as keratitis will cause true photophobia.

Glare

It is more likely that a patient complaining of sensitivity to light is being affected by glare and is not photophobic. Many people experience an increased sensitivity to glare as they age. Glare can be caused by sunlight, other lighting sources, and reflections from household sources.

There are two definitions of glare: **discomfort glare** and **disability glare**. With discomfort glare, the patient complains that the light within his or her visual field is excessively bright and is causing discomfort. There will be a higher level of luminance entering the eye to that currently adapted; the discomfort may impede functional performance.

The effect of disability glare is to impair the patient's visual performance. For example, a cataract may cause a scatter of light when there is high ambient illumination, and the eye will experience a drop in acuity.

In addition, **reflection glare** can occur to normal and visually impaired individuals when reading a shiny page of a book or magazine. The print is obscured: the angle of the incident light on the page and the (specular) reflected light entering the eye are equal. A shift in position of either the book or the reader will change the angle of either the incident beam or reflected light and the masking of the print is removed.

Management of photophobia and glare sensitivity

Management of the photophobia or glare sensitivity will focus on the underlying cause. For example:

- Treatment or removal of the underlying pathological cause.
- Removal or reduction of the light source or the scattered light.
- Change of position.
- Obstructing the light source: visors, shields, caps.
- Use of multiple pinholes.
- Typoscopes.
- Tints.

The use of reverse contrast print

Patients who suffer from photophobia or glare sensitivity tend to prefer reverse polarity of the print, when available. For example, in the use of a CCTV screen, all devices will provide the facility for reverse contrast. There is a significant reduction in the backscatter of light, which will improve the contrast of the retinal image.

Typoscopes (Fig. 7.6)

Typoscopes have the effect of reducing the backscatter of light in much the same way as using reverse contrast on a CCTV. Depending on the size of the hole, which is cut into the black card or sheet, one or several lines of print may be 'highlighted'. The typoscope additionally aids tracking and is often used in

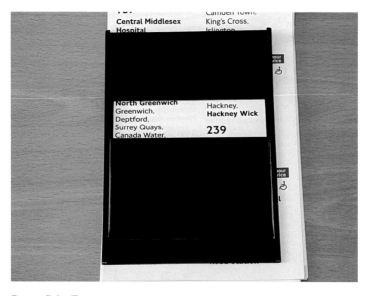

Figure 7.6 Typoscope

steady eye strategy. Patients who successfully use a typoscope often demonstrate improvement in reading performance. Some patients may tape a typoscope to the base of a stand magnifier.

Tints for glare

Any tint may be useful in bright sunlight, as sunglasses are useful on a sunny day. However, the degree of tint may impair visual function indoors or in levels of low illumination. Wrap-around sunglasses have the additional advantage of reducing unwanted sources from the sides (Fig. 7.7).

Photochromic lenses are often suggested as one of the better solutions to reduce the unwanted effects of discomfort glare. However, the usefulness of these lenses will be dependent on how effective their reactions are in both bright sunlight and dim indoor illumination. The lens reacts in response to UV radiation

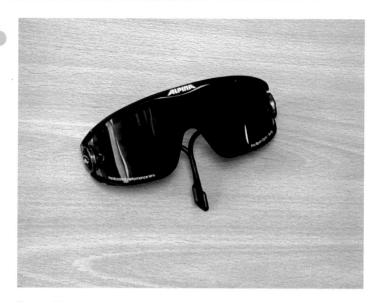

Figure 7.7 Wrap-around sunglasses

and will be less effective in high levels of artificial illumination, which may not suit some patients. However, for most, they can be quite useful.

The main objective when prescribing a tint for disability glare is to improve visual performance by selectively absorbing the scattered light and improving retinal image contrast. This is difficult to achieve with a tint, as it necessitates selective absorption characteristics of the tint. So it is not surprising that the tints give very mixed results, objectively and subjectively.

Some retinal disease (such as Stargardy's and retinitis pigmentosa) may benefit from specific orange/red tints.

Albinism and aniridia

There will be more light entering the eye in the case of patients with albinism or aniridia. Both will be affected by discomfort glare, and this is usually managed by the use of tints, especially out of doors. Both may additionally benefit from the use of contact lenses with an artificial pupil to reduce the amount of light entering the eye. Both conditions require normal or increased task lighting for near.

Cone dysfunction rod monochromatism

Patients often respond well to very dark filters. Performance improves in low levels of illumination, by using a tint of LTF (light transmission factor) 2–5%.

Lighting for low vision

Too much or too little light can be a problem for a person with low vision.

General lighting

With age, the amount of light entering the eye is reduced. Weale[63] suggested that there is a threefold drop in transmission between a 60-year-old compared to a 20-year-old eye. This can have the effect of reducing acuity, contrast perception and color discrimination.

The CIBS (1984) Code for internal lighting[76] recommends that illuminance levels for the elderly should be increased by 50–100%. However, several studies have shown that a large proportion of homes occupied by the elderly have illumination levels markedly below recommended levels. In some cases the poor levels of illumination will result in a reduced visual performance for many tasks.

Task lighting

Good lighting is important for performing near tasks such as reading. Patients with low vision benefit from increased task lighting.[77]

For example, the CIBSE (1984) Code recommends illuminance levels of 300 lux for sustained reading or sewing for younger patients. This would need to be increased to between 450 and 600 lux in elderly patients (>65) and significantly more, to approximately 1000 lux, in patients suffering from a visual impairment such as age-related macular degeneration.

The CIBS (1984) Code also recommends that the ratio of the task illuminance to that surrounding should not exceed 3:1. Therefore, large differences in light levels should be avoided both between the task and the rest of the background. Patients should be recommended to increase room lighting when they increase task lighting and to avoid using a bright lamp in a very dark room.

Color contrast

The importance of contrast perception was dealt with in Chapter 4. The use of color contrast in the home, however, in various daily living tasks has become widely used. For example, color contrast is used in the house and home as a practical approach to various recognition tasks. It improves the speed and accuracy of naming familiar objects and can be indispensable to many who live alone. A large number of devices distributed by the RNIB use color contrast successfully.

Examples of use

- *Bump-ons*. These are self-adhesive, raised tactile markers produced in a variety of bright colors, which may be used to highlight anything from cooker dials to switches.
- Colored buttons of various shapes may be sewn into clothing to aid identification.
- Patients may be advised to use colored items in the home, such as using a colored bar of soap against a white sink; tea or coffee is best served in a white mug and fish is easier seen on a dark colored plate.
- Colored masking strips may be used to demarcate the edges of internal obstacles, such as steps.

Using other senses

Auditory and tactile stimuli are used for both visually impaired patients and those with little or no sight. Devices produced may also be used in combination with other strategies such as high contrast definition, color contrast or relative size magnification.

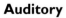

Auditory

The spoken word

Most libraries have access to a large range of books that have been produced in either casset or CD-ROM format. Interlibrary loan schemes are often available to widen the accessibility of the range of publications.

Calibre

Calibre is a registered charity, which was set up in 1974 to provide a postal lending library service to people who, for whatever reason, are unable to read ordinary print books. Calibre produces over 7000 titles, of which 1000 are suitable for children. All publications are recorded unabridged on ordinary cassets and the service is free.

The Talking Newspaper Association and Local Talking Newspapers

The Talking Newspaper Association of the UK (TNAUK) is a registered charity, which provides national and local newspapers and magazines on audiotape, computer disk, e-mail and CD-ROM for visually impaired and disabled people. Local newspapers and magazines are supplied free of charge by over 520 local talking newspaper groups which are affiliated to TNAUK but are autonomous.

The RNIB's Talking Books

The Talking Books service produced by the RNIB is the UK's main source of audio leisure reading. The service has over 70,000 members, and books are produced in several languages, with a choice of over 10,000 titles. The service is open to anyone who is registered as severely sight impaired or who can demonstrate acuity of N12 or less 'with best correction'. Annual membership is approximately £50.

Titles are produced in non-commercially available format. Initially produced in a non-standard casset format, books are now produced on a CD-ROM, called 'Daisy' books (Fig. 7.8).

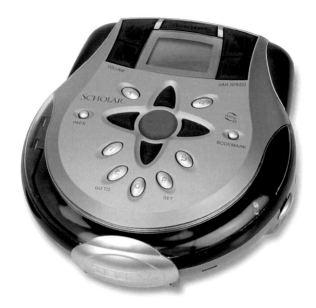

Figure 7.8 Scholar 'Daisy' Player

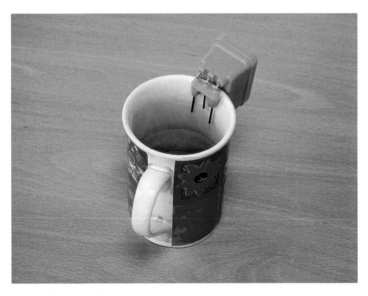

Figure 7.9 Liquid level indicator

Daily living equipment incorporating an auditory stimulus

Examples include:

- Liquid level indicators (Fig. 7.9).
- Talking watches and clocks.
- Talking tins (Fig. 7.10).
- Talking greeting cards.
- Talking microwave.

Tactile

Braille and Moon

Braille has been in use since Louis Braille first devised it in 1824. The English version consists of 63 symbols, which includes the

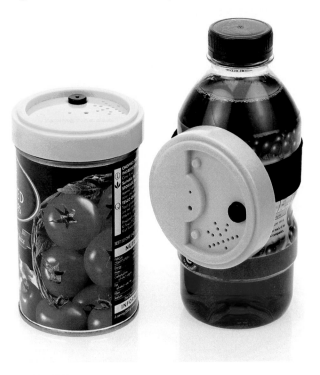

Figure 7.10 Talking tins

alphabet, punctuation and some letter combinations. It is more popular than Moon, which was also produced around the same time by Dr William Moon in 1845. The latter is based on a simplified form of the Latin alphabet and although it is simpler than Braille, being easier to use by those patients with less sensitivity in their fingertips, it is very bulky and slow to produce and, therefore, the uptake of readers is few.

The National Library for the Blind holds the largest source of books, which are available on loan. The RNIB also produces magazines, journals, cards, household items and personal items with Braille tactile indicators, and transcription services are readily available.

'Tacti-Mark'

'Tacti-Mark' is similar to Bump-ons. Also produced by the RNIB, it is a black fluid, which sets hard as a raised tactile marker, which can be used to mark various items.

8
Psychological factors in visual impairment

The longer one works in visual impairment, the more one realizes that much of the benefit for the patient is gained from having a knowledgable person listen to them and discuss their visual state with them. The importance of active listening and reassurance cannot be overemphasized. It is important, therefore, for the practitioner to be an adept communicator and also someone who is able to interpret the finer nuances of body language and non-verbal behavior in order to adequately meet the needsand expectations of the patient.

Nature of the vision loss

In Chapter 1, the definitions outlined in the ICIDH1 were described. It is common to find patients with similar impairments, say loss of central acuity, who are affected quite differently. In one the disability and resulting handicap may be great while the second patient through various coping strategies may find little handicap to their chosen lifestyle as a result of the impairment.

In general, the age of onset of the impairment has a major role in influencing the disability. Patients with congenital eye disorders have to adapt to their visual surroundings from the start of life and will develop a variety of strategies, some often most imaginative, in coping with everyday tasks. It is most heartening to examine a patient with a significant visual impairment who is finishing a degree or has just completed a major sporting or physical challenge.

Acquired sight loss is often less well adapted to and a brief glance at the epidemiology of sight loss (see Chapter 2) immediately highlights that the majority of visually impaired are elderly and most have lost sight through eye disease in mid-life (diabetes) or especially in later life (macular degeneration, cataract, glaucoma, etc). This presents a challenge to the patient in adapting to a new visual circumstance and it is essential for the practitioner to be able to understand this point.

A 70-year-old man may have happily read newspapers on his lap for many years and driven himself about. A sudden loss of acuity may result in both these tasks becoming either impossible or very difficult and a great deal of time and effort may be required for him to attempt to relearn tasks. An optometrist is a potentially very helpful professional in the rehabilitation of this man.

Factors other than age play a role, however, and it is too simplistic to assume that the longer a person has good levels of acuity before impairment occurs, the greater the disability. Factors include the people around the patient, environmental issues, the presence of other impairments, both physical and mental (secondary impairment is common in many visually impaired patients). This has been recognized in the later established ICIDH2 classification referred to in Chapter 1, and varying influences relating to the disability are specified.

A further factor is the perception of the impairment and its impact by the patients themselves which will be explained further later in this chapter.

Coping with loss

It is generally recognized that there are various stages in dealing with loss which most people to varying degrees pass through. This may be the loss of a partner, a limb or a sensory function.

The initial stages are often shock and denial of the impairment. Many a patient may refuse to accept that they are losing sight and will react in such a manner either to hide the impact or simply not believe there is any change in circumstance.

This eventually is not possible to maintain and the next stage is often anger at the fact that sight loss has occurred. Throughout both these stages calm and reasonable support is often useful, though generally speaking clinical and rehabilitative intervention is not appropriate nor will it be appreciated by the patient.

The next stage is often depression, when the patient has finally accepted that an impairment is there and feels disillusioned as to why it had to happen to them. An experienced practitioner may be some help at this stage in explaining the condition and outlining how, with a degree of effort and determination, there may be ways of coping with the impairment and preventing it from completely disrupting the lifestyle the patient had once taken for granted.

Eventually, and over a variable timescale between each individual, a patient comes to accept their lot and with this acceptance usually comes some degree of motivation to 'not be beaten' by the impairment. It is at this last stage that intervention and management is likely to be most effective.

Put yet more simply, an optometrist may have a role in empathizing, explaining and encouraging when a patient has yet to come to terms with their sight loss, and may help the patient who has accepted their loss by advising on relevant and achievable coping strategies.

Giving information

One of the commonest grievances described by the visually impaired relates to a lack of understanding of the actual nature of their disease. The fact that many patients learn most about their eye disease from the internet is a sad reflection of the fact that no eyecare professional has taken the time to explain the condition or spent time answering any questions. Most patients are able to cope better with their impairment if they understand it, can relate it to the visual deficit they perceive, and are aware of the potential for any future changes in their visual state. Sadly, too many people are still told that they 'have gone blind and there is nothing to be done' or, commonly with macular degeneration, that 'you will never go blind' despite the fact that the patient is no longer able to read or write.

An optometrist is ideally placed to give this sort of information and a few minutes spent in the consulting room explaining an eye disease to a patient is invaluable and genuinely appreciated. Much of this time is often spent dispelling various myths about disease. Patients arrive with a whole variety of health beliefs which will affect their motivation and ability to adapt. Often these are based on exaggerated anecdotes from friends and relatives about eye diseases, or sensationalist reports in the media. Again, the practitioner has a duty to put these in correct context.

Managing expectations

From the outset, a patient should be offered a realistic expectation of what might be achieved by the low vision assessment. Too many patients arrive in low vision services having been told that 'there is no treatment but go and see the optician for some strong glasses and this will improve things'. This is a disastrous start for the optometrist as often any attempt to use magnification will result in disappointment. Words such as 'improve' and 'make better' are best avoided. However, this does not mean that a negative attitude need be adopted and it is reasonable for the optometrist to describe how they are going to measure the vision a patient has and try and help them use it to better advantage. This still accentuates the positive without setting up unrealistic expectation.

Assessing motivation

If the first statement by the patient is 'there's nothing you can do for me' then it is a foolish practitioner who piles on the magnifiers. A good understanding of the patient's motivation should influence the management approach. In this case, a more useful plan would include some degree of counseling and regular visits to build up a rapport and to coax out details about the patient which may lead to them beginning to develop an ambition to cope differently with their impairment.

Often, poor motivation is not spoken of directly. The practitioner may detect a negative or defensive response pattern during the initial history taking. They may notice inappropriate responses during the assessment itself (for example, wildly changing acuity levels or the stated inability to read something which all the clinical evidence up to that point has indicated should be well within the patient's grasp).

It is important to remember, however, that apparently poor motivation may be part of the coping strategy of the patient and if they genuinely feel they cannot carry out a task such as reading then it would be foolhardy to force them to try. A much better approach is to be encouraging and open without being forceful or prescriptive.

Setting realistic goals

If an assessment is full of blurred and poorly interpreted targets, patient morale and, therefore, motivation is likely to plummet.

If, however, careful choice is made of task size, a real sense of achievement might be inculcated.

When deciding on a management plan for the less motivated patient (a well motivated patient will happily try anything), setting a simple goal within a set time scale is useful. Trying to watch television with eccentric viewing for 10 minutes a day until the next visit is perfectly possible. Often the patient will rise to the challenge if offered a 'get-out clause'. By stating that it will be difficult, and you fully expect at the next visit for the patient to tell you it was not possible, very often sows the seed of determination to prove you wrong. Furthermore, knowing they are going to see you again in a stated time (often, sadly, not possible in busy hospitals and resource centers) provides encouragement to attempt a set task.

Continued observation and contact is most useful not just for building motivation, but also in monitoring any change in circumstance and adapting the management plan accordingly. Vision may get worse still, a job might become impossible, or the patient may receive help from another source. All of these will affect the patient's ability to carry out your recommendations and ongoing monitoring will overcome this.

Responses: what the patients have to say

There are a number of frequent myths, misunderstandings and misinterpretations that can occur before, during or following the low vision examination.

'I need stronger ones'

Particularly on the first visit, many patients will attend a low vision consultation with a variety of ambitious ideas and expectations. Or, conversely, none at all. A previous practitioner may have told them, rather inappropriately, that the low vision practitioner can provide them with 'stronger glasses'. This is one of the most common and frustrating hurdles to overcome. 'Stronger glasses' come with a penalty. Often the considerably shorter working distance for some is difficult to overcome. A +20 diopter spectacle magnifier will have a working distance of 5 cm which, compared to a lifetime of reading a newspaper on a lap, may for some be particularly difficult to conquer.

'The more I wear them the worse it will get'

Due to failing sight, many patients may be trying not to use their glasses for fear of using up what little sight that they have left. It is often necessary to try to encourage patients that in using their glasses their vision will not deteriorate.

'Can I have a bigger one?'

Often it is difficult to explain that it is the smallest magnifiers that contain the stronger lenses. Patients returning with an aid frequently want one to cover the whole page, eliminating the need for continuously moving the magnifier over the paper and leaving one hand free. However, the practicalities of spectacle lenses are best explained at the outset and every attempt to achieve maximal field of view through the magnifier lens achieved at the start.

'But you told me I would never go blind'

It is not unusual for a patient to develop two visually impairing conditions at the same time. The ARMD may have stabilized, but a month later the patient is found to have glaucoma.

'But I want to read on my lap'

A reduced working distance is often a difficult hurdle to overcome, more particularly for those who have spent a lifetime with the paper on their lap. Those with an acquired loss regularly compare his/her sight to what it used to be. However, patients who have grown up with a congenital sight loss may be more accustomed to holding the object close.

These and many other problems have to be addressed before or during the eye examination. However, despite the frustrations there are still many who will come with absolutely no idea at all what to expect. Here, at least we can start with a blank canvas. Unfortunately, these patients are often those with the least amount of motivation.

There are no miracles to be found in the low vision consulting room. However, there is the occasional patient who we have helped way beyond their wildest expectations, frequently making a huge difference in their quality of life. And often, that perception alone is marvelous.

How useful the remaining vision is will depend on the patient's determination and level of expectation, what it is they want to see, and the circumstances in which they use it. Some patients will instinctively pick up an aid and use it. Some, despite increasing the magnification, may not achieve an improvement in VA. This often occurs in patients with a recent onset of macular degeneration and a central scotoma. On a consecutive visit they may appear to have a dramatic improvement in near VA. Eccentric viewing technique now mastered, the improved independence has all been worthwhile.

Total loss of sight is very rare indeed. Most people will retain some form of residual vision. To some, the loss will be devastating, to others a minor irritant. Patients who have lost sight to 1/60 often keep eye contact and will step over the toy box on their way into the consulting room. They are less likely to bump into things compared to someone with a gross visual field defect. Alternatively, the patients with a gross field defect may retain central vision.

The purpose of the low vision examination is to restore some quality of life to your patient. Remember that by far the majority of your patients are elderly, and may be rather nervous, possibly hard of hearing and often forgetful. If we work on the belief that two memories are better than one, it is usually helpful to have a friend or family member in the consulting room during the examination.

Communication tips

Some key points when communicating with a low vision patient:

- The practitioner needs to be sensitive to the patient's emotional response to their impairment, especially so in the case of an acquired impairment. Bearing in mind that the commonest cause of registerable blindness in the UK is age-related macular degeneration, it is not uncommon for a patient to have 70 years' worth of good functional vision which is lost over just a few months or years. In many cases, the first few LVA appointments may well deal primarily with advice and counseling to allow for some acceptance and rationalization of the situation before any care plan is embarked upon.

- The absence of external signs of the problem, combined with the general perception that blindness means total lack of visual function, often means that relatives and carers of the patient are less supportive than might be expected. The practitioner may play a useful role here.

- By setting realistic and achievable goals ('read for just 10 minutes a day with this magnifier until you can read the whole of the TV listing') is a simple yet effective way of increasing patient involvement in their care plan.

- The practitioner needs to remember that patients are not governed by ray diagrams and while an aid may be issued of the perfect magnification and best optical design, this is no guarantee that it is of any more perceived use to a patient than an old scratched magnifier given to them by a friend!

- When sight is an integral part of the communication process, such as with patients with an associated hearing impairment, there may be a need to develop a very flexible approach in patient management over a period of time.

- A patient is more than a pair of eyes. Any advice you offer needs to address this obvious fact and merely dishing out LVAs without understanding how someone might incorporate them into their daily life will result in disappointment for patient and practitioner alike.

Staff and environment

The physical environment is important. Many patients will find the visit to the practice an arduous and hazardous journey. This may be to the detriment of compliance and motivation. As well as accessibility issues, a practice should be designed such that mobility is not hindered. Well contrasting surroundings, uncluttered spaces and the absence of potential fall or trip hazards are all important. The environment is not just physical, however, and for the establishment of a good rapport with a patient, and therefore a well-motivated patient willing to take on board your advice, all members of staff need to be friendly, knowledgeable about visual impairment, and avoid stigmatizing or stereotyped attitudes. A degree of staff training in these areas is well worth the time and effort.

9
Community care, benefits and services

What is a low vision service?

> 'A person with low vision is someone who has an impairment of visual function for whom full remediation is not possible by conventional spectacles, contact lenses or medical intervention and which causes restriction in that person's everyday life.' (Low Vision Consensus Group, 1999)[3]

> 'A low vision service is a rehabilitative or habilitative process which provides a range of services for people with low vision to enable them to make use of their eyesight to achieve maximum potential.' (Low Vision Consensus Group, 1999)[3]

Essentially, a low vision service can be considered to be one of a number of services provided to people with a visual impairment. It includes the provision and training of low vision aids, to maximize the useful sight that a patient may still have. It further includes other non-optical low vision aids, the importance and correct usage of light and contrast enhancement and other modifications to the home, office, school and outside environment that will assist our visually impaired people within the community to live a more fulfilling life.

Our Better Vision[2] researched the needs of UK based service users with regards to low vision services. It found that the delivery of effective low vision services is a positive experience for the vast majority of people, with the provision of low vision aids, training and support considered to be invaluable.

Low vision services reduce the disabling impact that serious sight problems can have by helping people make the most of their sight. A lack of low vision services will mean more residential care and rising costs for local authorities.[78] Therefore, in order to provide a comprehensive service to patients, it is sensible to become aware of low vision services provided at a local level, and how a patient can attain access to them. This is particularly important for those patients we are unable to deal with effectively within the consulting room. Working with patients with visual impairment is as much the giving of advice and information, as it is dispensing of a low vision device.

The report *Fragmented Vision*[78] presented quantitative research undertaken by the RNIB and Moorfields Eye Hospital in 1999, and concluded that the provision of low vision services in the United Kingdom was unacceptably poor in three fundamental areas: accessibility, distribution and delivery. Significantly, the report found that in some parts of the country where prevalence of low vision was high, there were no services at all. There was a lack of communication and joint working between different agencies and professionals delivering low vision services.

Services are often provided by a large number of different agencies:

- Health services.
- Social services.
- Voluntary sector and national charitable organizations.

Effective communication between the various groups and professional bodies involved in the provision of services is essential to provide consistency across the country. This is particularly true, given the large number of professionals involved in service provision. Ryan and Culham[78] found as many as 31 different professionals were involved in the provision of low vision services and low vision aids. These included:

- Optometrists.
- Dispensing opticians.
- Rehabilitation workers.
- Ophthalmologists.
- Specialist teachers.
- Social workers.
- Orthoptists, counselors, nurses.

Low Vision Consensus Group

In 1999 the **Low Vision Consensus Group** published the report: *Low Vision Services: recommendations for future service* *delivery in the UK.*[3] It recommended that a Local Low Vision Services Committee should be established in each area to ensure the delivery and quality of services. It further recommended the local integration of ophthalmic and rehabilitative care and support services. To make effective use of these services, people with low vision would need to be informed that the service exists, how to access the service, and would also need to know the standard of service they expect to receive. The report was widely endorsed as being a forward plan for the improvement of services across the country.

Local low vision services committees

Following the recommendations from the Low Vision Consensus Group, local low vision services committees are continuing to be set up around the country, in most cases, quite successfully. These committees are now considered to be the forum within which a local scheme and protocol should be drawn up and agreed.[4] Key stakeholders who will normally be represented on the local committee are:

- Service users.
- The primary care trust.
- Ophthalmology departments.
- The local optical committee.
- Community optometrists and dispensing opticians.
- Social services' teams for visual impairment.
- Voluntary organizations.
- General medical practitioners within the Primary Care Trust.

Locally based practitioners are now actively encouraged to involve themselves in the provision of low vision services. In most cases, the practitioner may need to undertake a training program prior to approval. The College of Optometrists Low Vision Group provides advice and recommendations for practitioners involved in locally based schemes.

The provision of low vision aids

At a local level, there are two main sources of information:

1. The Primary Care Trust/Local Health Authority

The Primary Care Trust will have a list of local providers of low vision aids. Access to this list can be gained by contacting the section leader of the ophthalmic division.

2. RNIB directory of low vision services in the UK

This service has been produced in association with Moorfields Eye Hospital NHS Trust and is available online from the RNIB website: http://info.rnib.org.uk.

Nationally there are numerous sources:

Hospital Eye Service (HES)

Most low vision aids are still supplied by the hospital eye service on a loan basis without charge. In some eye departments, this may be in association with a local voluntary organization. It is not necessary to be certifiable as blind or partially sighted to gain access to low vision clinics, but the individual will need to be a current hospital patient and thus will be referred through the GP in the usual way.

Historically, and perhaps inappropriately, many patients were left until their vision had stabilized, or reached the 'end of the road' until they were referred for low vision aid assessment. However, with improved education and communication between practitioners with different professional backgrounds, the provision of low vision aids has become more accessible even for those who are waiting for a routine cataract operation, or who are still awaiting treatment. Preferably, the service is made available to all patients at their point of need.

Optometrists manage most hospital low vision aid assessments. In some eye departments, a dispensing optician or an orthoptist may also provide low vision aids.

General Ophthalmic Services (GOS)

In the absence of a convenient clinic the ophthalmologist may issue an authorization for the patient to consult a local GOS optometrist or dispensing optician who will prescribe low vision aids on behalf of the hospital. There are also some optometrists/dispensing opticians who provide private services.

University optometry departments

Most of the UK optometry and dispensing departments provide a service, although some clinics may be limited to academic teaching time. They usually accept self-referrals, or referrals from the GP, Rehabilitation worker, etc. A full list of university departments is given in Chapter 11.

Voluntary sector provision

Many voluntary organizations, both national and local, provide low vision aids. These may be on a loan basis or in association with the Primary Care Trust (PCT). The PCT will typically have a list of low vision aid providers. Alternatively, the RNIB directory will be able to provide a local based search online.

CCTV provision and other specialist equipment

CCTVs are not available on loan from the Hospital Eye Service. The Local Education Authority (or Unitary Authority) will provide special equipment including CCTVs to schoolchildren following an assessment through Special Educational Needs.

Similarly, equipment can also be provided through the Access to Work (AtW) scheme to employees, if the need has been established through an assessment.

It is otherwise difficult to get a CCTV for home use through any other means. Some charities provide CCTVs and computer software products, although funds are often limited and products expensive.

Rights to community care services

Duties placed on Primary Care Trusts come under the National Health Service and Community Care Act (1990). It is important to note that it is not necessary to be registered as either blind/severely sight impaired or partially sighted/sight impaired in order to receive help through community care legislation. If the PCT accepts that there is a 'need', then help can and must be provided. Community care legislation is based on a government white paper, 'Caring For People'. This states that anyone who has problems with, for example, a mental illness, a learning disability or a physical disability should be able to obtain care services and support which *enables them to live in their own home and to retain as much independence as possible'*. These include, for example:

- Practical help and adaptations in the home.
- Training and special skills.
- Outside recreational facilities and a means of transport.
- Occupational therapy.
- Meals at home, etc.

A home visit and assessment takes place and a detailed care plan is established to meet these needs. The assessment will include a discussion of the unusual difficulties caused by poor sight, from identifying the controls on the cooker to fears about crossing the road, checking sell-by dates, or checking if the washing has been done. The assessment is not restricted to visual problems, and will take into consideration other factors such as physical disabilities or hearing impairment.

During the needs assessment, the visiting rehabilitation worker may go through some of the following recommendations:

- Color contrast.
- Lighting.

- Eccentric viewing.
- Reminding them how to use the magnifiers that they may have already been given.
- Encouraging the use of large print.
- They may demonstrate the Eezee-Reader.
- Demonstrating equipment that may make life easier.
- Large button telephones and arranging free directory enquiries service.
- Clocks, watches, scales and calculators.
- Writing frames, pension book guides, signature guides, envelope guides.
- Large-print bank statements, coin holders.
- Identifying bank notes.
- Liquid level indicators which bleep.
- Small self-adhesive tactile raised markers known as 'bump-ons' placed on cooker, washing machine and other controls.
- Large-print labels for tins and packets.
- Advice on home safety and in the garden.

Following the assessment and the care plan, a care manager is appointed as the individual who is responsible for bringing the whole range of different services together to meet the person's individual and unique needs. The care program will be monitored, as the patient's needs change. If a patient's needs have recently changed, and if it has been a while since the Social Services Department has assessed their needs, then it would not seem inappropriate to suggest that they have another assessment.

After the assessment there is a duty to provide. Some Social Services Departments have varying degrees of interpretation of 'need' and all have complete discretion to adopt any criteria they wish. Provision would typically cover daily living skills, communication and mobility training, recreational and social activities. However, all aspects of Primary Care Trust activity are often constrained by limited resources, and are also frequently understaffed. There is often a shortage of specialist workers, with some areas being better off than others.

Sometimes a service will be needed that the PCT cannot supply, e.g. mobility training. If the need for mobility training is accepted, then the trust has a duty to provide it and thus will buy in the services from elsewhere.

Certification and registration is not required

Under the Community Care Act (1990), a patient is entitled to services if they can demonstrate that they have a need. This is irrespective of certification or registration. However, patients are often not aware that they are entitled to a full assessment of their needs without the need for registration with the Primary Care Trust. Local optometrists are encouraged to give the patient the Letter of Vision Impairment (LVI 2003) to aid reducing the delay for assessment.

Furthermore, it has been well known that there has often been a delay between certification and registration. Therefore, the use of the Referral of Vision Impaired Patient (RVI 2003) by hospital clinic staff will also ensure that the assessment of needs is undertaken independent of certification and registration and, therefore, will help to reduce delays.

An RNIB study (1991)[43] found that, of those patients certified and registered as either blind or partially sighted, only 29% had received expert advice on entitlements, and only 1% had received practical advice on daily living skills. Furthermore, more than one-third of patients could not name a voluntary organization. However, the study also demonstrated that those who were registered were significantly more better informed than those disabled by their visual impairment, but who were not included on a PCT register. Within the past few years, there has been a greater emphasis on the local authorities to improve services.

Hearing and the visually impaired

There is usually someone based at Social Services who is responsible for people with a dual loss and who can communicate manually. Young people who have a congenital hearing loss are encouraged to get their sight tested regularly. Usher syndrome is widely misdiagnosed and often goes unrecognized.

Financial benefits

Certification and registration is, therefore, not required to obtain help and assistance from the PCT. However, registration is mandatory when claiming financial benefits. Registration is also often necessary when applying for many other benefits and concessions. Filling in the forms is a major undertaking. The 28-page self-assessment form is long. Questions are intimate, describing how the disability affects everyday life, and many people may find the procedure humiliating. The greatest danger is that at a quick glance they feel that the humiliation is easily avoided if the benefits are not pursued.

Where to access information
- In Touch (BBC web pages are by far the best source).
- Citizens advice bureau.
- RNIB helpline: 0845 766 9999.
- Welfare rights officers at local Social Services Departments.
- Benefits enquiry line: 0800 88 22 00.

There is no such thing as a 'blind pension', but there is a mixture of modest financial help, which can be triggered by registration.

A list of benefits is given in Table 9.1. The list is not exhaustive and is accurate at the time of printing. This list is frequently updated and can be viewed online at http://info.rnib.org.uk.

Travel concessions

Local concessions

Concessionary travel and the way it is delivered has changed dramatically over the last few years. Integration, flexibility, accessibility, quality and value for money have become important issues for local authorities in meeting the needs of a growing population of senior citizens and disabled users.

The Transport Act 2000[79] states that a registered disabled person, including those on the blind and partial sight registers, is entitled to receive a free half-fare bus pass for services within the area that he/she lives.

Table 9.1 Benefits and concessions for the blind and partially sighted

Name	Description	Blind	PS	Further information
Additional income support or pension credit	Tops up a low income. If 60 or over, claim pension credit	✓	✓	Income support: contact local Jobcenter pension credit: 0800 28 1111
Blind person's personal income tax allowance		✓		
Disability living allowance (DLA) or attendance allowance (AA)	For help with personal care and mobility. Claimed before 65. Those aged 65 and over claim AA	✓	✓	Contact local social security office or Benefit enquiry line on 0800 88 22 00
Additional housing benefit or Council Tax		✓	✓ (Only if the person gets DLA or AA)	Contact local council housing benefit or Council Tax benefit sections
Exemption from 'non-dependants' deduction from Income Support,		✓	✓ (Only if the person gets DLA or AA)	

Continued

Table 9.1 Benefits and concessions for the blind and partially sighted—cont'd

Name	Description	Blind	PS	Further information
Pension credit, Housing benefit and Council Tax benefit				
Council Tax reduction		✓	✓	Contact local Council Tax section about the reductions for people with disabilities
Incapacity benefit	For people of working age who are incapable of work	✓	✓	Contact local social security office or ring the Benefit Enquiry line 0800 88 22 00
Working tax credit	For disabled people on low incomes working at least 16 hours per week	✓	✓	Tax credit helpline on 0845 300 3900
Help towards residential or nursing home fees	Financial help towards residential or nursing home costs may be available	✓	✓	Contact local council social services department or Benefit Enquiry line on 0800 88 22 00

Service			Details	Contact
Community care services and assistance from local council	✓	✓	Services include home care, mobility training, counseling, equipment or home adaptations	Contact your local council social services department
Free NHS sight test	✓		Also available to anyone over 60	Local optometrist
Free NHS prescriptions	✓	✓	Depends on age and income. Those unable to go out without help may also be eligible	Ask RNIB Welfare Rights Service for details
Low vision aids	✓	✓		RNIB Eye Health Unit for further information. Call 0845 766 9999 or local optometrist
Reduction in television license fee	✓		Registered blind people get 50% reduction on the standard rate	Call the television license helpline on 0870 576 3763 for further information
Car parking concessions under the Blue Badge Scheme	✓		The car doesn't need to be yours	Contact social services. Partially sighted people must show they have problems walking

Continued

Table 9.1 Benefits and concessions for the blind and partially sighted—cont'd

Name	Description	Blind	PS	Further information
Special equipment, a reader or assistance at work and help with travel costs	Provided under the Access to Work Scheme	✓	✓	Details from Jobcenters or RNIB Employment Network: 0845 766 9999
Free postage on items marked 'articles for the blind'	Braille or recordings like Talking Books. Not personal tapes and letters	✓	✓	
Railcard and other rail travel concessions		✓	✓	Contact local railway station, or call RNIB/GDBA Joint Mobility Unit on 020 7388 1266
Local travel schemes		✓	✓	Contact local council for details of travel concessions
Exemption from BT Directory Enquiry charges		✓	✓	Ring 195 and ask for a PIN number

| Free permanent loan of radios, casset players and TV sound receivers | British Wireless for the Blind Fund | ✓ | Contact local council social services department |
| Help with telephone installation charges and line rental | 'Telephones for the Blind Fund' | ✓ | Contact local council social services department |

Information source: RNIB, 2003

Although all local authorities must now offer a half-fare bus pass, many also offer transport tokens as an alternative. The Department for Transport has further confirmed that token schemes may work alongside the half-fare bus pass as laid down in the Transport Act 2000.

The advantage of token schemes is that the tokens can be used to provide a choice of travel for those people who live where there are inadequate bus services or who have a disability which prevents them from using a bus—or simply for those people who prefer to retain the flexibility to choose their own form of travel.

National travel concessions

The disabled persons railcard
Entitles discount for national rail travel.

Wales
Free concessionary travel for pensioners and disabled people on buses.

Scotland
National free travel scheme
Holders of a Scottish Blind Persons Travel Card are entitled to free travel (standard class) on:

- All local bus services in Scotland.
- All express bus services in Scotland.
- All rail services in Scotland.
- Glasgow underground services.
- Ferry services.

Private coach companies
Some operating long distance will give concessions.

Domestic flights
- In certain circumstances, some concessions are available on inland flights by domestic airlines.
- Anyone traveling by air will receive help at the airport provided they contact the airport in good time.

10
Education and employment

Education

The Government's Green Paper[79] followed on from the Code of Practice on the identification and assessment of special educational needs[80] in promoting mainstream classroom placement for all children.[81]

There are an estimated 23,000 children with a visual impairment in the UK, with one in three being identified as having multiple disabilities and a visual impairment (Table 10.1).[82] These additional disabilities include impaired hearing or speech, physical handicaps or learning difficulties; 9000 of these are in primary school.[83] Fifty-three percent of children with a visual impairment attended a local mainstream school in 1988 and this figure rose to 59% in 1995.[83,84]

The recent draft revised code of practice on the identification and assessment of special educational needs[80] states that 'there is a clear expectation within the Education Act 1996, that pupils with special educational needs will be included in mainstream schools...the Government believes that when parents want a mainstream place for their child the education service should do everything possible to try and provide it.'[81]

A survey by the RNIB[85] estimated that there are a total of 10,000 children in Great Britain with a visual impairment severe enough to pose problems at school. Although relatively small in number compared with the total number of visually impaired, children represent a lot of 'patient years'. The survey also showed the struggle that parents have to obtain information and advice about their child's condition. Special counseling was shown to be rare, yet nearly three-quarters of parents said that they would have welcomed it.

Education options[83,84]

Local mainstream	53%
Mainstream with resource base	6%
Special school for visual impairment	10%
Other special schools	29%
Other, e.g. independent home tutoring	2%

Table 10.1   Numbers of children registered by March 2003

Scotland 31st March 2003		
	Age 0–5	Age 6–15
Blind	93	332
PS	45	364
England 31st March 2003		
	Age 0–4	Age 5–17
Blind	725	3230
PS	525	4230

All visually impaired children are encouraged to make maximum possible use of their vision in whatever type of education they are in, whether they are being educated in a special or a mainstream school. The aim is to enable them, wherever possible, to learn by sighted methods. Many children are now in mainstream schools with support from a classroom assistant or support teacher. Good optical assessment and provision is, therefore, essential if this aim is to be achieved.

Children Act 1989[88]

This Act, which covers many aspects of the rights, welfare and education of children, states that:

- Help should be available to all 'children in need'.
- A child is considered 'in need' if he is 'unlikely to achieve or maintain, or to have the opportunity of achieving or maintaining, a reasonable standard of living'.
- Registration as Blind/PS by the local authority/PCT is therefore not necessary to establish a 'need' under the Children Act.

It has been suggested that 23,000 people under the age of 19 have impaired vision, with less than 1000 using Braille.[82,84]

Therefore, we could assume that the vast majority will have some measurable functional vision, who will require optometric services, or at least regular low vision assessments. This becomes particularly important when a child becomes introduced to print.

Special educational needs (SEN)

Local education authorities (LEAs) employ educational advisers or peripatetic teachers or visually handicapped children who are knowledgable in child development and learning and are able to offer expert help to mothers of preschool and school age children. These are known as qualified teachers of the visually impaired (QTVI).

LEAs have a duty to identify, assess and provide for all children recognized with special educational needs from the age of two.[88] Before this, the responsibility lies with the local social services or local child health services under the instruction of the PCT.

Disability Rights Commission

The Disability Rights Commission (DRC) has been set up to work towards the elimination of discrimination against disabled people. From September 2002, the Disability Discrimination Act 1995 (as amended by the Special Educational Needs and Disability Act 2001) will make it unlawful for providers of education and related services to discriminate against disabled people.[86]

Under the 1996 Education Act, schools and education authorities are required to provide help to visually impaired children. When a child embarks on their education, the Primary Care Trust must inform the LEA of any child who is likely to have Special Educational Needs. The child need not be registered Blind or Partially Sighted at this stage, but the LEA notification is mandatory from the age of 2 and up to the age of 19.

In the case of newly diagnosed children, the GP will first refer the child to a children's developmental unit for a comprehensive assessment of the child's needs. The team there may include a pediatrician, educational psychologist, physiotherapist, occupational therapist and a social worker. The assessment process should provide the basic information on which a program of education and treatment can be based, and also refers the parents to appropriate sources of help outside the unit.

Once a child has been identified as having special needs, there is then a five-stage code of practice during which a Special Educational Needs Coordinator (SENCO), together with the LEA, may request assessments from outside specialists. All schools have a SENCO, usually the head teacher (or deputy head teacher), who is responsible for special educational needs in the school.

With visually impaired children, these additional assessments and reports may be requested from the child's ophthalmologist and hospital optometrist (if he or she has one). Other reports may also be requested from an educational psychologist, or the child's GP, etc. Once reports have been put together, the LEA will consider the child's needs and produce a written statement (in Scotland: Record of Needs). This written document will outline the child's needs for special equipment, such as low vision aids or a CCTV, transport to school, or perhaps the extra tuition from a specialized teacher or the inclusion of a classroom assistant, etc. In the case of the visually impaired child, it is important that mobility and keyboard skills are also included. Once this fifth stage has been reached it is typical to have an annual review. Parents are actively involved in this process.

Once something has been detailed in the statement, then there is a duty for the LEA to provide it.

Mainstream education

If a child remains within mainstream education, additional support is often provided. The nature of provision varies widely between LEAs. Additional help may be provided within the classroom by teaching assistants or may be provided by specialist teachers (QTVIs) for the visually impaired. The latter may choose to withdraw the child at some stages to a designated unit and cover, for example, the teaching of Braille, mobility skills, tactile skills and keyboard skills. However, inclusion in the main activities taking place in the classroom is crucial for improving access to the curriculum and developing the child's skills of social interaction and independence, especially those children with a severe impairment, who may require additional support in developing social and life skills.

Employment

For visually impaired people either seeking a job, or for those who are having difficulty at work as a consequence of their impairment, help both to the employee and employer is obtainable from the Department for Work and Pensions.

Disability Employment Advisers

Disability Employment Advisers (DEAs) are normally based at job centers around the UK. DEAs are members of Disability Services Teams (DSTs). They can provide help to people with a disability who are looking for employment, or additional employment support for those whose disability is starting to affect them within work. Following a comprehensive interview, the DEAs will typically draw up an action plan for the individual.

In addition, they may:

- Offer advice and support to help improve the job prospects of people with disabilities.
- Arrange for assessment services to help secure appropriate work or training. This can include a low vision assessment to identify whether special workplace aids or equipment are needed.
- Arrange for visually impaired people to attend residential and non-residential employment rehabilitation courses.

Access to Work[87]

Access to Work (AtW) is a program that provides practical support to both disabled people and their employers to overcome difficulties in the workplace resulting from a disability. Help may include, for example, special equipment, a support worker, a communicator, alterations to premises and help towards travel to work costs if unable to use public transport. This is achieved by paying a grant, through job centers, towards the costs needed to provide the additional support.

The visually impaired person who needs additional equipment at work, for example, a CCTV, will initially make contact with the nearest AtW business center. The AtW adviser will contact the employer and a meeting may often take place within the workplace. In the case of CCTV, the adviser will arrange for a CCTV assessment. Typically, the employer will obtain the equipment and then claim back the grant from the AtW (Table 10.2).

The grant is often a percentage of the total cost of the approved support, although up to 100% may be claimed in some circumstances, although this is usually dependent on the length of time the individual has worked for the employer.

All help is over a maximum of 3 years, after which the AtW business center will review the support.

'Work preparation'

This is an individually tailored program helping individuals prepare for employment by identifying and overcoming any barriers that they may have, usually via a period of work placement with an employer. Residential programs for people with visual impairments are available, although most programs are run as near as possible to home.

Table 10.2 **Costs as outlined by Department for Work and Pensions, July 2004**

Approved cost	Maximum AtW contribution
Less than £300	Nil
Between £300 and £10,000	80% of the cost over £300
Over £10,000	80% of the cost between £300 and £10,000 and 100% of the cost over £10,000

'Workstep'

Previously known as supported employment, Workstep provides job support to over 26,000 disabled people who face more complex barriers to getting and keeping a job, but who can work effectively with the right support. It enables eligible disabled people to realize their full potential to work within a commercial environment, giving them, whenever possible, an opportunity to progress into open employment. The program also offers practical assistance to employers.

11
Some useful information sources

Action for Blind People
14–16 Verney Road, London SE16 3DZ, United Kingdom.
Tel: +44 20 7635 4800
http://www.afbp.org/homepage.htm

Action for Blind People enables blind and partially sighted people to transform their lives through work, housing, leisure and support. They offer a wide range of services to visually impaired people, their families, advocates, professionals and the general public. Among these services are:

- Practical employment development support for visually impaired people and companies.
- Support for blind and partially sighted people wishing to move home and specialist housing units.
- Four purpose-built and specially adapted hotels for visually impaired guests.
- A national information and advice service, with specialized welfare rights support.

Beacon Centre for the Blind
Wolverhampton Road East, Wolverhampton, West Midlands, WV4 6AZ, United Kingdom.
Tel: +44 1902 880111
http://www.beacon4blind.co.uk

The Beacon Centre is totally independent of any other charitable organization offering services to the blind. In existence since 1875, they currently provide services for several thousand registered blind and partially sighted people living in Wolverhampton, Dudley, Sandwell and South Staffordshire. Facilities include a residential home for the blind, specially adapted bungalows, a day center, after-school club, domiciliary visiting service, supported business, mobile resource unit, hospital information desk, carer support and a toy library.

Bord Athshlanuchain
(National Rehabilitation Board)
44 North Great George Street, Dublin 1, Ireland.
Tel: +353 1 874 7503
Email: nrb@iol.ie

British Council for Prevention of Blindness (BCPB)

12–14 Harcourt Street, London W1H 4HD, United Kingdom.
Tel: +44 20 7724 3716
http://www.bcpb.org

Their mission is to prevent blindness and restore sight in the UK and the developing world by:

- Funding research in UK Hospitals and Universities into the causes and treatment of the major eye diseases.
- Supporting practical treatment programs and research in the developing world.
- Promoting vital skills, leadership, awareness and demand for community eye health in the developing world through the education of doctors and nurses.

British Retinitis Pigmentosa Society

PO Box 350, Buckingham, Buckinghamshire, MK18 5EL,
United Kingdom.
Tel: +44 1280 860363 (Helpline); +44 1280 860195 (Office)
http://www.brps.demon.co.uk

The Society is a membership organization run by volunteers with over 35 branches throughout the UK. It aims to provide a better understanding of the inherited retinal disorders known as retinitis pigmentosa (RP), macular degeneration, Usher syndrome and other allied retinal dystrophies. The BRPS raises funds for scientific research and provides a welfare support and guidance service to its members and their families.

Calibre

New Road, Weston Turville, Aylesbury, Bucks.,
HP22 5XQ, United Kingdom.
Tel: +44 1296 432 339
Fax: +44 1296 392 599
http://www.calibre.org.uk

Calibre is a registered charity, set up in 1974 to provide a postal lending library service to people who, for whatever reason, cannot read ordinary print books. The service is free to members—we do not charge a subscription—so we rely on *help* to maintain and expand the service. We have over 19,500 members, and offer a choice of 7000 titles to borrow, of which some 1000 titles are suitable for children. All recorded unabridged on ordinary cassets. The books are delivered by post and the service is free.

Christian Blind Mission (CBM)
Winship Road, Milton, Cambridge CB4 6BQ,
United Kingdom.
Tel: +44 1223 426161
http://www.cbmuk.org.uk/home.shtm

CBM is an association of committed Christians dedicated to serving eye patients, blind and otherwise disabled people in the developing world, irrespective of nationality, race, gender or religion. The work of CBM centers around medical care, curing and preventing blindness, as well as the rehabilitation and training of disabled people and their integration into society: helping people to help themselves.

Deafblind UK
National Centre for Deafblindness, John and Lucille van Geest Place, Cygnet Road, Hampton, Peterborough PE7 8FD, United Kingdom.
Tel: +44 1733 358 100
Fax: +44 1733 358 356
http://www.deafblind.org.uk

Deafblind UK is currently assisting thousands of deafblind or dual sensory impaired people throughout the country to cope with their disability and to lead as fulfilled and independent lives as possible. Deafblind UK offers comprehensive services to deafblind people, their support assistants and other professionals. These include training in communication and rehabilitation skills, a free 24-hour help line, a regional network of staff and volunteers, a varied leisure program and a range of publications.

Guide Dogs for the Blind Association (Head Office)
Hillfields, Burghfield Common, Reading, Berkshire, RG7 3YG,
United Kingdom.
Tel: +44 118 983 5555

Fax: +44 118 983 5411
http://www.gdba.org.uk

The Guide Dogs for the Blind Association provides guide dogs, mobility and other rehabilitation services that meet the needs of blind and partially sighted people. The Association shapes its services to meet the needs of its community. While guide dogs are central to their work, they also provide practical living skills training such as reading and writing as well as other forms of mobility, for example, long-cane training—often in partnership with local authorities.

Guide Dogs funds work into ophthalmic and canine research, investing in new technology that could enhance the lives of the UK's blind and partially sighted population.

International Association for the Education of Deafblind People (IAEDB)

c/o SENSE, 11–13 Clifton Terrace, Finsbury Park, London N4 3SR, United Kingdom.
Tel: +44 20 7272 7774
Fax: +44 20 7278 6012
http://www.sense.org.uk

Activities: World and European conferences every 4 years. Biannual magazine: *Deafblind Education.* Staff development center. Committees on staff development, Usher syndrome, congenital deafblindness, acquired deafblindness, and communication.

International Centre for Eye Health

Department of Epidemiology & International Eye Health, Institute of Ophthalmology, University College London, 11–43 Bath Street, London EC1V 9EL, United Kingdom.
Tel: +44 20 7608 6907
Fax: +44 20 7250 3207
http://www.ucl.ac.uk/ioo

Activities: Courses in community eye health in London (MSc., Diploma, Certificate, short modules); establishment and continued support of international training centers. Provision of resources to international training centers. Consultancies for prevention of blindness agencies and national programs.

International Federation of Guide Dog Schools for the Blind (IFGDSB)

Hillfields, Burghfield Common, Reading, Berkshire, RG7 3YG, United Kingdom.
Tel: +44 118 983 1990
Fax: +44 118 983 3572
http://www.ifgdsb.org.uk

The International Federation of Guide Dog Schools for the Blind (IFGDSB) was formed in 1989, following meetings over several years of Guide Dog schools around the world. The IFGDSB now comprises 63 member schools around the world whose purpose is to serve the visually impaired through the breeding, training and provision of Guide Dogs.

International Glaucoma Association

King's College Hospital, Denmark Hill, London SE5 9RS, United Kingdom.
Tel: +44 20 7737 3265
Fax: +44 20 7436 5929
http://www.iga.org.uk

The IGA is a registered charity, which offers advice and support to glaucoma sufferers, campaigns for improved glaucoma services for glaucoma patients and aims to increase public awareness of glaucoma. They also fund considerable clinical research into the nature and treatment of the condition.

Membership of the IGA is open to patients, optometrists, opticians, doctors and all those interested in preventing loss of sight from glaucoma.

Jewish Blind & Disabled

164 East End Road, Finchley, London N2 0RR, United Kingdom.
Tel: +44 20 8883 1000
Fax: +44 20 8444 6729
http://www.jbd.org

Jewish Blind & Disabled provides caring sheltered housing for visually and physically disabled people, to help them improve their quality of life, maximize their freedom of choice, and achieve independent living.

Macular Disease Society
Darwin House, 13a Bridge Street, Andover,
Hampshire, SP10 1BE, United Kingdom.
http://www.maculardisease.org/

The Macular Disease Society is a self-help society for those suffering from any of the eye conditions encompassed by the overall name of 'macular disease'.

National Federation of the Blind of the United Kingdom
Chapel House, South Heighton, New Haven,
Sussex, BN9 0JH, United Kingdom.
Tel: +44 1273 514344
Fax: +44 1273 612691
http://www.nfbuk.org/

The NFBUK campaigns for better community care and rehabilitation services for all blind and partially sighted people, better access to buildings, improved transport facilities, better access to printed material, obstruction-free pavements and a whole number of other issues of concern to blind and partially sighted people.

National League of the Blind
59 Kinefold House, York Way Estate, York Way,
London N7 9QD, United Kingdom.
Tel: +44 20 7607 4794
Fax: +44 20 7388 0508
http://www.istc-tu.org

The National League of the Blind & Disabled (NLBD) is an independent trade union of disabled people formed in 1899 and affiliated to the TUC in 1902 and the Labour Party in 1909. It merged with the ISTC in February 2000 under a Transfer of Engagements which allowed the NLBD to continue its activities in

terms of Structure—Branches—Regional Councils—National Committee, affiliations in the Disability Movement and policy making machinery through a National Conference.
(Last updated: 20/02/2001)

National Library for the Blind (NLB)
Far Cromwell Road, Bredbury, Stockport SK6 2SG, United Kingdom.
Tel: +44 161 355 2000
Fax: +44 161 355 2098
http://www.nlb-online.org/

The National Library for the Blind provides a wide range of library and information services for visually impaired people, their families and anyone with an interest in visual impairment. It is a gateway to free comprehensive library services for all those who cannot read print and their intermediaries. Its aim is to enable all visually impaired people to have the same access to library services as sighted people. As well as lending a wide range of reading material for all age groups from its extensive collection of hard copy Braille and Moon books and Braille music, NLB also provides access to electronic books and reference material via its website.

National Listening Library
12 Lant Street, London SE1 1QR, United Kingdom.
Tel: +44 20 7407 9417
Fax: +44 20 7403 1377
http://www.listening-books.org.uk

Listening Books is a charity that provides audio books in casset format via the post to people who suffer from an illness or disability, which makes it impossible or difficult to hold a book, turns its pages, or read in the usual way. The service is available to institutions such as hospitals, residential and nursing homes and schools, as well as to individuals. They also provide support for the National Curriculum.

ORBIS International
2nd floor, 17 Islington High Street, London N1 9LQ, United Kingdom.

Tel: +44 20 7278 5528
Fax: +44 20 7278 5231
http://www.ukorbis.org

ORBIS is an international charity dedicated to eliminating avoidable blindness by training local doctors and medics in the developing world in vital sight-saving techniques. Training programs are held on board the ORBIS Flying Eye Hospital, a fully converted DC-10 jet (equipped with operating theater and classrooms), and in local hospitals and clinics in the developing world. In addition to the Flying Eye Hospital, ORBIS runs land-based teaching programs in Bangladesh, China, Ethiopia, India and Vietnam. ORBIS relies heavily on its volunteers who are medical professionals from the UK and other nations who give up their time to train local doctors and nurses in the developing world. With their assistance, ORBIS has held programs in over 80 countries and has trained over 50,000 doctors and nurses who, in turn, have treated over 15 million people worldwide.

Partially Sighted Society
Queen's Road, Doncaster, South Yorkshire, DN1 2NX, United Kingdom.
Tel: +44 1302 323132

The Partially Sighted Society was formed in 1973, mainly by parents of partially sighted children. Registered as a charity, it has grown into a nationwide organization having a national office, Sight Centers in Exeter and Wrexham, a London Regional Office, and nearly 30 branches throughout Great Britain.

Queen Alexandra College
Court Oak Road, Harborne, Birmingham B17 9TG, United Kingdom.
Tel: +44 121 428 5050
Fax: +44 121 428 5048
http://www.qac.ac.uk

Queen Alexandra is a national residential college providing assessment, rehabilitation, further education and vocational training for adults with a visual impairment and/or other disabilities. Also, QAC Enterprises is a wholly owned subsidiary of Queen Alexandra College offering professional Braille and audio production, and engineering services.

Royal Blind School

Craigmillar Park, Edinburgh EH16 5NA, United Kingdom.
Tel: +44 131 667 1100
Fax: +44 131 662 9700
http://www.royalblindschool.org.uk/

The Royal Blind School is a day and residential school with a long tradition in the education of pupils with visual impairments. The school is based at two sites, both on the south side of Edinburgh. The largest site is the Craigmillar Park Campus where the pre-school unit, primary and secondary schools are based. The second site at Canaan Lane houses a unit for pupils with visual impairments and profound and complex learning difficulties.

Royal London Society for the Blind (RLSB)

Dorton House, Seal, Nr Sevenoaks, Kent, TN15 0ED, United Kingdom.
Tel: +44 1732 592500
Fax: +44 1732 592506
http://www.rlsb.org.uk/

The Royal London Society for the Blind is committed to empowering people with a visual impairment to lead independent lives through the provision of high quality education, training and employment services. Established in 1838, the Royal London Society for the Blind (RLSB) is one of the oldest charities set up to look after the needs of blind and partially sighted people. Today, the RLSB provides a range of vital services to support people who are visually impaired. The Society is a national and international provider of education, training and employment opportunities for people who are visually impaired.

Royal National College for the Blind

College Road, Hereford HR1 1EB, United Kingdom.
Tel: +44 1432 265725
Fax: +44 1432 353478
http://www.rncb.ac.uk

The RNC is the UK's largest College of Further Education and training for people who are blind or partially sighted. Programs include: employment assessment and work preparation, GCSEs, A/AS levels, access to HE, remedial therapy, performing arts, art and design, music technology, information technology, business studies, piano technology, and administration.

Royal National Institute of the Blind (RNIB)
105 Judd Street, London WC1H 9NE, United Kingdom.
Tel: 0845 766 99 99 (UK callers only)
Tel: +44 20 7388 1266 (Switchboard/Overseas callers)
Fax: +44 20 7388 2034
http://www.rnib.org.uk

The RNIB exists to promote the better education, training, employment and welfare of blind people, to protect their interests and to prevent blindness.
   (Last updated: 05/12/2002)

Royal National Institute for the Deaf (RNID)
19–23 Featherstone Street, London EC1Y 8SL,
United Kingdom.
Tel: +44 808 808 0123
Fax: +44 20 7296 8199
http://www.rnid.org.uk

The Royal National Institute for Deaf People (RNID) is the largest charity representing the 9 million deaf and hard of hearing people in the UK.

Mission: To be a powerful force for change with government, and public and private sector organizations; to change radically the attitudes and behavior of individuals towards deaf and hard of hearing people; to provide services directly to deaf and hard of hearing people to improve their everyday lives; to be a catalyst for research in medicine and technology to improve the lives of people with a hearing loss; and to seek to work in partnership with those who share our vision and mission.

Royal School for the Blind
Church Road North, Wavertree, Liverpool L15 6TQ,
United Kingdom.

Tel: +44 151 733 1012
Fax: +44 151 733 1703
http://www.rsblind.org

The Royal School for the Blind provides places for up to 66 pupils ranging in age from 2–19 years. All students have a visual impairment and learning difficulties ranging from moderate to profound. Many students have additional sensory, physical or behavioral disabilities.

Scottish Braille Press
Craigmillar Park, Edinburgh EH16 5NB, United Kingdom.
Tel: +44 131 662 4445
Fax: +44 131 662 1968
http://www.scottish-Braille-press.org

Printers and publishers of Braille and producers of audio, large print and tactile diagrams.

Scottish Sensory Centre
Moray House Institute of Education, Holyrood Road, Edinburgh EH8 8AQ, United Kingdom.
Tel: +44 131 651 6402
Fax: +44 131 651 6502

The Scottish Sensory Centre promotes and supports new developments and effective practices in the education of children and young people with sensory impairments: visual impairment, deaf and deafblind.

SeeABILITY
SeeABILITY House, Hook Road, Epsom, Surrey, KT19 8SQ, United Kingdom.
Tel: +44 1372 755000
Fax: +44 1372 755001

SeeABILITY is a registered charity, working with adults who are visually impaired and have additional disabilities (learning disability, physical disability, degenerative conditions, mental health difficulties), supporting them to explore their potential, develop their skills/independence and/or enhance the quality of their lives.

Services offered include: assessment, visual impairment rehabilitation, day care, research, supported living and residential and nursing care services. Additionally, consultancy and training services are offered to carers/other professionals.

SENSE
11–13 Clifton Terrace, Finsbury Park, London N4 3SR,
United Kingdom.
Tel: +44 20 7272 7774
Text: +44 20 7272 9648
Fax: +44 20 7272 6012
http://www.sense.org.uk

SENSE is one of the leading national voluntary organizations supporting and campaigning for deafblind people, their families, supporters and professionals who work with them. Sense offers advice, help and information to deafblind people and their families; supports families through a national network and local branches; runs a holiday program for deafblind children and adults; provides education, residential, respite and day services; has communicator-guides and one-to-one intervener support; offers training and consultancy.

Sightsavers International (The Royal Commonwealth Society for the Blind)
Grosvenor Hall, Bolnore Road, Haywards Heath,
West Sussex, RH16 4BX, United Kingdom.
Tel: +44 1444 446663
Fax: +44 1444 446677
http://www.sightsavers.org.uk

Sightsavers International is the UK's leading charity working to prevent the tragedy of needless blindness in developing countries and to bring hope to people who will never see again. Sightsavers International works in over 20 countries in Asia, Africa and the Caribbean.

St. Dunstan's Caring for Blind Ex-Service Men and Women
12–14 Harcourt Street, London W1H 4HD, United Kingdom.

Tel: +44 20 7723 5021
Fax: +44 20 7262 6199
http://www.st-dunstans.org.uk

St. Dunstan's provides training, rehabilitation and lifelong aftercare for blind ex-service men and women and their families.

St. Vincent's School for Blind and Partially Sighted Children

Yew Tree Lane, West Derby, Liverpool L12 9HN,
United Kingdom.
Tel: +44 151 228 9968
Fax: +44 151 228 5266
http://www.stvin.com

St. Vincent's is a non-maintained school of charitable status offering both day places and weekly boarding. The school is approved by the Department for Education and Employment, with a long and successful tradition, dating back to 1850, of education and care for blind and partially sighted children.

Talking Newspaper Association of the UK (TNAUK)

10 Browning Heathfield, East Sussex, TN21 8DB,
United Kingdom.
Tel: +44 1435 86 9310
http://www.tnauk.org.uk/

The Talking Newspaper Association of the UK (TNAUK) is a registered charity, which provides national and local newspapers and magazines on audiotape, computer disk, e-mail and CD-ROM for visually impaired and disabled people who find reading a strain. Local newspapers and magazines are supplied free of charge by over 520 local talking newspaper groups which are affiliated to TNAUK but are autonomous.

A 'Guide to Tape Services for Visually Impaired and Disabled People' is available from TNAUK in print and on disk and contains details of **local talking newspaper** groups, other information available on tape and organizations for visually impaired and disabled people.

Tiresias
http://www.tiresias.org

This website is an information resource for professionals who work in the field of visual disabilities. The site has evolved from work carried out by Dr Janet Silver of Moorfields Eye Hospital, London, and Dr John Gill of the Royal National Institute of the Blind.

Torch Trust for the Blind
Torch House, Hallaton, Leicestershire, LE16 8UJ, United Kingdom.
Contact person: Michael Stafford, General Administrator
Tel: +44 870 7700 272
Fax: +44 870 7700 262
http://www.torchtrust.org

The Torch Trust for the Blind is a non-denominational Christian charity that provides Christian literature and fellowship for visually impaired people. Literature is produced in Braille, large print (24 pt) and on audiocasset and they operate a free postal library service, including a children's and young people's section, for all three media. Torch is also an international ministry with bases in Malawi and Romania, and is in touch with blind people in over 90 countries of the world.

**Wales Council for the Blind
(Cyngor Cymru i'r Deillion)**
3rd Floor, Shand House, 20 Newport Road, Cardiff CF24 0DB, Wales.
Tel: +44 29 2047 3954
Fax: +44 29 2043 3920
http://www.wcbnet.freeserve.co.uk

WCB is the leading Welsh organization in the field of visual impairment, working with a network of voluntary and statutory agencies to improve provision for people with sight problems in Wales.

UK Universities and Colleges

The Department of Optometry,
School of Biomedical Sciences,
University of Ulster,
Coleraine.
Co. Londonderry, BT52 1SA,
Northern Ireland.
Tel: +44 (0) 2870 324 891
Fax: +44 (0) 2870 324 965

Department of Optometry,
University of Bradford,
Richmond Road,
Bradford.
West Yorkshire, BD7 1DP.
Tel: +44 (0) 1274 235567
Fax: +44 (0) 1274 235570

The Department of Optometry and Neuroscience,
UMIST,
Sackville Street,
Manchester M60 1QD
Tel: +44 (0) 161 200 3870
Fax: +44 (0) 161 200 4433

Department of Optometry & Ophthalmic Dispensing,
School of Applied Sciences,
Anglia Polytechnic University,
East Road,
Cambridge CB1 1PT.
Tel: +44 (0) 1223 363271
Fax: +44 (0) 1223 417712

Department of Optometry and Visual Science,
City University,
Fight for Sight Optometry Clinic,
7–9 Bath Street,
London EC1V 0HB.

Tel: +44 (0) 20 7040 8339
Fax: +44 (0) 20 7040 8494

Department of Vision Sciences,
Glasgow Caledonian University,
70 Cowcaddens Road,
Glasgow G4 0BA.
Tel: +44 (0) 141 331 3000
Fax: +44 (0) 141 331 3005

Optometry and Vision Sciences,
School of Life & Health Sciences,
Aston University,
Aston Triangle,
Birmingham B4 7ET.
Tel: +44 (0) 121 359 3611
Tel: +44 (0) 121 333 4220

School of Optometry and Vision Sciences,
Cardiff University,
Redwood Building,
King Edward VII Ave.,
Cathays Park,
Cardiff CF10 3NB,
Wales.
Tel: +44 (0) 29 2807 4374
Fax: +44 (0) 29 2807 4859

Association of British Dispensing Opticians
199 Gloucester Terrace,
London W2 6LD.
Tel: +44 (0) 20 7298 5100
http://www.abdo.org.uk

Association of Optometrists
61 Southwark Street,
London SE1 0HL.
Tel: +44 (0) 20 7261 9661
Fax: +44 (0) 20 7261 0228
http://www.assoc-optometrists.org

College of Optometrists
42 Craven Street,
London WC2N 5NG
Tel: +44 (0) 20 7839 6000
Fax: +44 (0) 20 7839 6800
http://www.college-optometrists.org

Federation of Ophthalmic and Dispensing Opticians
199 Gloucester Terrace,
London W2 6LD.
Tel: +44 (0) 20 7298 5151
Fax: +44 (0) 20 7298 5111
http://www.fodo.com

General Optical Council
41 Harley Street,
London W1N 2DJ.
Tel: +44 (0) 20 7580 3898
Fax: +44 (0) 20 7436 3525
http://www.optical.org

For information regarding the Certificate of Visual Impairment (2003)
Janet Goodwin
Disability Policy Branch,
Room 544, Wellington House,
133–155 Waterloo Road,
London SE1 8UG.
Email: Janet.Goodwin@doh.gsi.gov.uk
Tel: +44 (0) 20 7972 4121
Website information: http://www.dh.gov.uk

References

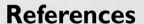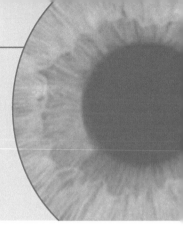

1. RNIB: Estimates and Registration Statistics for the UK, 1995.
2. Ryan, B. and McCloughlan, L. (1999). *Our better vision: what people need from low vision services in the UK.* London: RNIB.
3. Low Vision Consensus Group (1999). *Recommendations for future service delivery in the United Kingdom.*
4. Framework for a Multidisciplinary Approach to Low Vision (2001). The College of Optometrists.
5. WHO, Geneva (1980). *International Classification of Impairments, Disabilities and Handicaps.* pp. 25–31.
6. Shuntermann, M.F. (1996). *The International Classification of Impairments, Disabilities and Handicaps (ICIDH)—results and problems.* Int J Rehab Res **19**:1–11.
7. Speech by Dr Gro Harlem Brundtland, Director-General, World Health Organization at WHO Conference on Health and Disability, April 2002.
8. BD8 Record of Examination to certify a person as blind or partially sighted. London: HMSO.
9. Form No. BP1 (2R) issued by The Scottish Office Home and Health Department, St Andrew's House, Edinburgh.
10. Form A655. Northern Ireland.
11. CVI (2003). Explanatory Notes Version 1, 6 Nov. 2003, Department of Health.
12. *Bye Bye BD8.* Richard Cox, Course Director, RNIB School of Rehabilitation Studies (2003).
13. Evans, J.R. and Wormald, R.P.L. (1993). *Epidemiological function of BD8 Certification.* Eye **7**:172–179.
14. CVI (2003). Department of Health.
15. Foster, A. and Johnson, G.J. (1990). *Magnitude and causes of blindness in the developing world.* Int Ophthalmol **14**:135–140.
16. Vision 2020 The Right to Sight. The Global Initiative for the Elimination of Avoidable Blindness. World Health Organisation, Feb. 2000.
17. Wormald, R. *Epidemiology of Macular Disease: World and UK Statistics, Risk Factors and Socio-economic Impact of AMD.* Elizabeth Thomas Seminar on Macular Degeneration; University of Nottingham Royal College of Ophthalmologists Congress, 2001.

18. Owen, C.G., Fletcher, A.E., Donoghue, M.D. and Rudnicka, A.R. (2003). *How big is the burden of visual loss caused by age related macular degeneration in the United Kingdom?* Br J Ophthalmol **87**(3):312–317.

19. Evans, J. (1995). *Causes of blindness and partial sight in England and Wales, 1990–1.* Office of Population Consensuses and Surveys. Studies on medical and population subjects. London: HMSO.

20. Population figures from General Blind and Partial Sight Register Office, Scotland.

21. Northern Ireland Health and Social Services Board (31/3/94). Belfast: NIHSSB, 1994.

22. Registered blind and partially sighted people: year ending 31 March 2003, England. 12 December 2003. Source: SSDA 902 form, Department of Health.

23. Shaw, C. (1998). 1996-based national population projections for the United Kingdom and constituent countries. Population trends.

24. Snellen, H. (1862). *Scala Tipografica Measurae il Visus* (Utrecht).

25. Rumney, N. J. (1995). *Using visual thresholds to establish low vision performance.* Ophthal Physiol Optics **15**(Suppl 1):18–24.

26. Thomson, D. (2003). Chapter 1: The assessment of vision. In Doshi S, Harvey W, *Investigative Techniques and Ocular Examination.* Butterworth-Heinemann.

27. Bailey, I.L. and Lovie, J.E. (1976). *New design principles for visual acuity letter charts.* Am Optom Physiol **53**:740–745.

28. Heron, G., Furby, H.P., Walker, R.J., Lane, C.S. and Judge, O.J.E. (1995). *Relationship between visual acuity and observation distance.* Ophthal Physiol Opt **15**(1):23–30.

29. Gilchrist, J. (1996). *Bias and precision of letter chart threshold estimates: a simulation study.* Ophthal Physiol Opt **16**(3):254.

30. Pierscionek, B.K. and Weale, R. A. (1999). *A logistics evaluation of visual acuity as applied to the Bailey–Lovie chart.* Ophthal Physiol Opt **19**(6):507–511.

31. McMonnies, C.W. (1999). *Chart construction and letter legibility/readability.* Ophthal Physiol Opt **19**(6):498–506.

32. McMonnies, C.W. and Ho, A. (2000). *Letter legibility and chart equivalence.* Ophthal Physiol Opt **20**(2):142–152.

33. Thomson, D. (2003). *Use and development of computer based test charts in the assessment of vision.* Chapter 2 in *Investigative Techniques and Ocular Examination.* Butterworth-Heinemann.

34. Whittaker, S.G., Lovie-Kitchen, J.E. (1993). *Visual requirements for reading.* Optom Vis Sci **70**:54–65.

35. Regan, D. and Neima, D. (1983). *Low contrast letter charts as test of visual function.* Ophthalmology **90**:1192–1200.

36. Arden, G.B. (1988). *The importance of measuring contrast sensitivity in cases of visual disturbance.* Br Ophthalmol **62**:198–209.

37. Legge, G.E., Ross, J.A., Luebker, A. and LaMay, J.M. (1989). *Psychophysics of reading. VIII. The Minnesota low-vision reading test.* Optom Vis Sci **66**:843–853.

38. Baldasare, J., Watson, G.R., Whittaker, S.G. and Miller-Shaffer, H. (1986). *The development and evaluation of a reading test for low vision individuals with macular loss.* J Vis Impairm Blindness **80**:785–789.

39. Watson, G.R., Wright, V., De l'Aune, W., Long, S. (1996). *The development and evaluation of a low vision reading comprehension test.* J Vis Impairm Blindness **90**:486–494.

40. Legge, G.E., Ross, J.A., Maxwell, K.T. and Luebker, A. (1989). *Psychophysics of reading VII. Comprehension in normal and low vision.* Clin Vis Sci **4**:51–60.

41. Ahn, S.J. and Legge, G.E. (1995). *Printed cards for measuring low-vision reading speed.* Vis Res **35**:1939–1944.

42. Mansfield, J.S., Ahn, S.J., Legge, G.E. and Luebker, A. (1993). A new reading-acuity chart for normal and low vision. *Ophthalmic and Visual Optics/Non-invasive Assessment of the Visual System Technical Digest, (Optical Society of America, Washington, D.C., 1993)* **3**:232–235.

43. Bruce, I., McKennell, A. and Walker, E. (1991). *Blind and Partially Sighted adults in Britain: the RNIB Survey, Vol. 1.* London: HMSO.

44. Wolffsohn, J.S. and Cochrane, A.L. (2000). Design of the low vision quality of life questionnaire (LVQOL) and measuring the outcome of low vision rehabilitation. Am J Ophthalmol **130**:793–802.

45. Wolffsohn, J.S., Cochrane, A.L. and Watt, N.A. (2000). *Implementation methods for vision-related quality-of-life questionnaires.* Br J Ophthalmol **84**:1035–1040.

46. Community Care Act 1990. London: HMSO.

47. Legge, G.E., Rubin, G.S., Pelli, D.G., Schleske, M.M. (1985). *Psychophysics of reading II. Low vision.* Vision Res **25**:253–266.

48. Arden, G.B. (1978). *The importance of measuring contrast sensitivity in cases of visual disturbance.* Br J Ophthalmol **62**:198–209.

49. Arden, G.B. (1988). *Testing contrast sensitivity on clinical practice.* Clin Vis Sci **2**:213–224.

50. Bailey, I.L. (1978). *Visual acuity measurement in low vision.* Optom Monthly (April), 116–122.

51. Bailey, I.L. (1993). *New procedures for detecting early vision losses in the elderly.* Optom Vis Sci **70**:299–305.

52. Brown, B. (1981). *Reading performance in low vision patients; relation to contrast and contrast sensitivity.* Am J Optom Physiol Opt **58**:218–226.

53. Bullimore, M.A. *Face recognition image-related maculopathy.* Invest Opthalmol Vis Sci **32**:2020–2029.

54. Grey, C.P. and Yap, M. (1987). *Edge contrast sensitivity in optometric practice: an assessment of its efficacy in detecting visual dysfunction.* Am J Optom Physiol Opt **64**:925–928.

55. Leat, S.J. and Woodhouse, J.M. (1993). *Reading performance with low vision aids; relationship with contrast sensitivity.* Ophthal Physiol Opt **13**:9–16.

56. Pelli, D.G. and Robson, J.G. (1987). *The design of a new letter chart for measuring contrast sensitivity.* Clin Vis Sci **2**:187–199.

57. Culham, L. (1983). *Training low vision patients.* Optician **200**:11–15.

58. Cummings, R.W., Whittaker, S.G., Watson, G.R. and Budd, J.M. (1985). *Scanning characteristics and reading with a central scotoma.* Am J Optom Physiol Opt **62**:833–843.

59. Fletcher, D.C., Schuchard, R.A. and Warren, M.L. (1993). *A scanning laser ophthalmoscope preferred retinal locus scoring system compared to reading speed and accuracy.* Invest Ophthalmol Vis Sci **34**:787.

60. Goodrich, G.L. and Quillman, R.D. (1977). *Eccentric viewing training.* J Vis Imp Blind **71**:377–381.

61. White, J.M. and Bedell, H.E. (1990). *The oculomotor reference in humans with bilateral macular disease.* Invest Opthalmol Vis Sci **31**:1149–1161.

62. Bailey, I.L. (1983). *Can prisms control eccentric viewing?* Optom Monthly **74**:360–382.

63. Weale, R.A. (1961). *Retinal illumination and age.* Trans Illum Eng Soc **26**:95–100.

64. Boyce, P.R. (1973). *Age, illuminance, visual performance and preference.* Lighting Res Technol **5**:125–144.

65. Eldred, K.B. (1992). *Optimal illumination for reading in patients with age-related maculopathy.* Optom Vis Sci **69**:46–50.

66. Lehon, L.H. (1980). *Development of lighting standard for the visually impaired.* J Vis Imp Blind **75**:249–253.

67. Sloan, L.L. (1969). *Variation in acuity with illuminance in ocular diseases and anomalies.* Docum Opthamol **26**:384–393.

68. Sloan, L.L., Habel, A. and Feiock, K. (1971). *High illumination as an auxiliary reading aid in diseases of the macula.* Am J Ophthalmol **76**:745–757.

69. Norville UK. Ophthalmic lens catalogue.

70. Genensky, S.M., Petersen, H.E., Moshin, H.L., Clewett, R.W. and Yoshimura, R.I. (1972). *Advances in closed circuit TV systems for the partially sighted*, Rand R-1640-HEW/RC.

71. Genensky, S.M., Petersen, H.E., Moshin, H.L., Clewett, R.W. and Yoshimura, R.I. (1972). *Advancements in closed circuit television systems for the partially sighted.* Santa Monica: Rand R-1040. HEW/RCA.

72. Genensky, S.M. (1969). *Some comments on a closed circuit TV system for the visually handicapped.* Am J Optom **46**:519–524.

73. Schreier, E.M.*, Levanthal, D.D., Uslan, M.M. (1991). *Access technology for blind and visually impaired persons.* Technol Disabil **1**(1):19–23.

74. Harvey, W.J. (2004). *Electronic low vision aids, a new image for the visually impaired.* Optician **227**(5948), April 23rd.

75. http://www.eyecare-information-service.org.uk

76. CIBS (1984). Code for internal lighting, 5th Edition. London: The Chartered Institution of Building Services Engineers, Lighting Division.

77. Rosenberg, R. *Illuminating Solutions: Tips for Lighting and Low Vision.* Educational Publications, Lighthouse International. Updated (2003) by Rosenthal, B., Faye, E. and Lloyd, S.

78. Ryan, B. and Culham, L. (1999). *Fragmented Vision. Survey of Low Vision Services in the UK.* RNIB and Moorfields Eye Hospital Trust.

79. Department for Education and Employment (1997). *Excellence for All Children: Meeting Special Educational Needs.* London: HMSO.

80. Department for Education and Employment (2000). Draft revised Code of Practice on the Identification and Assessment of Special Educational Needs. London: HMSO.

81. Davis, P. (2002). *Including Children with a Visual Impairment in Mainstream Primary School Classrooms.* Presentation given at International School, Psychology Association Annual Colloquium, Nyborg.

82. Clunies-Ross, L., Franklin, A. and Keil, S. (1999). *Blind and Partially Sighted Children in Britain: Their incidence and special needs at a time of change.* RNIB for the Nuffield Foundation. London.

83. Clunies-Ross, L. and Franklin, A. (1997). *Where have all the children gone?* Br J Vis Impairm **15**:48–52.

84. Walker, E., Tobin, M. J. and McKennel, A. (1992). *Blind and partially sighted children in Britain: the RNIB survey,* Vol. 2. London: HMSO.

85. Blind and Partially Sighted Children in Britain. RNIB survey 1992.

86. Disability Discrimination Act 1995 as amended by the Special Educational Needs and Disability Act 2001. London: HMSO.

87. http://www.jobcentreplus.gov.uk

88. Children Act 1989. London: HMSO.

Index